CHINESE
HOME REMEDIES

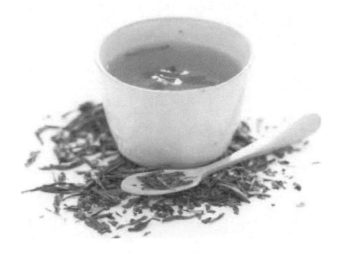

*Harnessing Ancient Wisdom
for Self-Healing*

Lihua Wang, L.Ac.

 *New Page Books
A division of The Career Press, Inc.
Franklin Lakes, NJ*

CHINESE HOME REMEDIES
Cover design by Cheryl Cohan Finbow
Printed in the U.S.A. by Book-mart Press

To order this title, please call toll-free 1-800-CAREER-1 (NJ and Canada: 201-848-0310) to order using VISA or MasterCard, or for further information on books from Career Press.

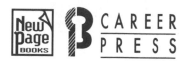

The Career Press, Inc., 3 Tice Road, PO Box 687,
Franklin Lakes, NJ 07417
www.careerpress.com
www.newpagebooks.com

Library of Congress Cataloging-in-Publication Data

Wang, Lihua.
    Chinese home remedies : harnessing ancient wisdom for self-healing
(including an A to Z listing of ailments and their remedies) / by Lihua Wang.
        p. cm.
    Includes index.
    ISBN 1-56414-808-4 (pbk.)
    1. Medicine, Chinese. 2. Medicine, Popular. I. Title.

R601.W32197 2005
601'.951--dc22

                                                                2005041559

Dedication

DEDICATED TO THE MEMORY
OF HOLLY TSHINLI YAP BLIATOUT.

Acknowledgments

I would like to thank Martin Stadius, a great writer and friend, for his indispensable editorial help on the manuscript.

Many thanks to Jean Dugan, Sandra Profeta, Carin McCameron, and Odell Hoffmann for reading the manuscripts and offering great suggestions.

Thanks to the editors at New Page Books and my agent Joanne Wang for their support throughout the entire process of writing this book.

My mentors and colleagues in China had a profound impact on my development in medicine. While it is impossible to list them all, I would like to especially thank Prof. Wang Mian Zhi and Prof. Liu Du Zhou of Beijing College of Traditional Chinese Medicine for nurturing me in the art of healing.

My former colleagues and students at Oregon College of Oriental Medicine have helped me on countless occasions. I am deeply indebted to them.

Finally, this book would not have been possible without the generous spirit and inspiring examples of my patients over the years. In this book, I have tried to instill the knowledge and skills that I have gained while treating and listening to them. They are the true parents of this book. I wish to express my most profound gratitude to them for allowing me the opportunity to accompany them through their journey of healing.

A Word of Caution

This book is intended as a reference only, not as a medical manual. Most of the home remedies herein are based on prolonged experimental practices. But medical science is constantly developing and changing, and, therefore, the reader should always consult a medical doctor before trying any home remedies contained in the text. Also the constitution of each individual is different and complex. Some remedies may be good for one person while ineffective for another. Use one remedy for three to five days unless otherwise indicated. Many of the treatments described in the book are not intended for pregnant women unless otherwise indicated. The Chinese herbs in this book are for reference only. All the remedies that involve Chinese herbs should be taken with consultation with professional herbalists. Also, the patent herbs mentioned in this book are not necessarily the best choices; they are listed because they are most available in the United States.

This book mentions a variety of substances such as herbs, herbal cream, and vegetables to be applied on skin. They may cause an allergic reaction. Therefore, whenever you want to use such treatment, do a skin test first. Apply the substance on a penny-size patch of your skin. Wait for 24 hours, and if there is an allergic reaction, stop using it. Don't use herb wine remedies if your health situation is not suitable to take alcohol, such as fever, hemorrhagic disease, cancer, hepatitis, respiratory disease, and so on.

Note

ALL THE HOME REMEDIES HEREIN ARE BASED ON PROLONGED EXPERIMENTAL PRACTICES. THE AUTHOR HAS MADE EVERY EFFORT TO MAKE ALL THE INFORMATION CORRECT. MEDICAL SCIENCE IS CONSTANTLY DEVELOPING AND CHANGING, THEREFORE THE AUTHOR AND PUBLISHER ARE NOT RESPONSIBLE FOR ANY OMISSIONS AND MISTAKES THAT MAY BE FOUND IN THE TEXT, OR ANY ACTIONS THAT MAY BE TAKEN BY A READER AS A RESULT OF ANY RELIANCE ON THE INFORMATION CONTAINED IN THE TEXT.

Contents

PART TWO:
SELF-HEALING WITH TRADITIONAL CHINESE MEDICINE
HOME REMEDIES A TO Z
33

APPENDIX:
WHERE TO GET CHINESE HERBS,
PATENT HERBS, AND SPECIFIC ITEMS

Foreword

When I was a young girl growing up in Beijing, my grandmother lived with us. She had simple home remedies for every ailment in the household. I was often amazed how effective they were. The kitchen was her pharmacy. Ingredients such as pepper, vinegar, sesame oil, ginger, and even pears became her medicine.

I still remember the horror of finding acne appearing on my cheeks as a teenager. My grandma told me to rub saliva on the breakout. I thought her idea was strange, but followed her advice. To my surprise, the developing sores faded away. I asked Grandma how it worked. She said, "I don't know. It just works." Actually, she didn't have an answer for most of her remedies.

Later in my life, I attended the College of Traditional Chinese Medicine and studied both Western medicine and Chinese medicine. I discovered that some of Grandma's methods might have had a basis in science.

For example, acne is caused by excess oil clogging skin pores. The salivary glands secrete an enzyme called lipase, which digests fat and oil molecules. The acne was digested by saliva. I thought yeast might be more powerful because it has more digestive enzymes. I used yeast whenever I got acne during those stressful school years, and the acne disappeared.

My brother often had nosebleeds as a child. My grandma had him hook his index fingers together and pull as a nosebleed began. The nosebleed almost immediately ceased. I thought a possible mechanism for this treatment was the tension in the body caused by the hooked fingers might affect the blood dynamics.

I collected these home remedies in my third year of college because I realized that they would be helpful in my future medical career.

In 1979, I was a physician practicing both Western and Chinese medicine at the Academy of Traditional Chinese Medicine in Beijing, and was sent to a remote village near the Yellow River to act as a barefoot doctor.

This is one of the poorest areas in China, where the arid soil yields very little harvest. The peasants worked hard but still couldn't earn enough to put food on the table. Of course, they couldn't afford healthcare. When they had a disease, they depended on the folk remedies and village shaman.

I once saw a villager who had eczema-like symptoms on his forearm. His mother said it was caused by damp toxin, which needed fire-based treatment. She carefully stripped a piece of cotton to its thinnest possible layer, down to a translucent film. She put it over the affected area and touched it with a lighted match. The cotton film burst in flames and quickly burned itself out. The man only felt a flash of warmth. But I would advise against using this method as a home remedy because of the inherent danger of fire. The next day, the eczema-like problem was gone.

I realized that the villagers treated their own illnesses with material they had on hand, generation after generation. Their experiences were so valuable, but (I found) were not written anywhere. While I did my best to heal people with very limited medical resources, I started to record all the folk remedies I could find. I shouldered a bag for collecting herbs and traveled through the mountain villages, stopping everywhere to talk to the locals about their traditional cures. I wrote down everything I saw and heard among the villagers.

When I returned to my hospital in Beijing, I applied these remedies on my patients whenever the opportunity arose.

In 1988, I came to America to treat patients and teach at the Oregon College of Oriental Medicine. In 1992, I started my own private practice. I have utilized these remedies, and continued to refine them. I've seen a wide variety of ailments in my patients. Some of them had tried and exhausted all treatments. Often, after they followed my advice on living healthier and tried my simple home remedies, the chronic problems that plagued them for years were resolved.

My decision to write this book is intimately related to my own experience.

Last year, I had a very mild injury to my right hand. The next morning, I awoke up with an extreme burning pain in that hand, which had become purple, and my fingers had swollen like sausages. I was diagnosed as having Reflex Sympathetic Dystrophy Syndrome (Complex Regional Pain Syndrome). It is a rare disease with few treatments available. The sufferers usually experience terrible pain on a daily basis, and some of them become permanently disabled. I re searched this condition and was devastated. A few days later my bones started to enlarge. At that time, I thought my life as I knew it was finished. Even as I contemplated many dark thoughts, I began to treat myself, attacking the disease with all the power of home remedies I had gained over the years. It was the simple, folk-based remedies that proved effective against this devastating illness. Soon, much to everyone's surprise, the pain lessened and I was regaining the function of my hand. Eventually, I emerged from the disease without taking one painkiller or becoming disabled.

For all the years I've practiced medicine, this was the first time I experienced, personally, how a debilitating disease can wreak havoc on a person's life and family. I thought countless others and their families could benefit from my knowledge. It was my duty as a human being to spread my knowledge about home remedies to others, and this book is the result of my efforts.

I have written this book in the hope that my experiences both as a patient and healer can help and inspire sufferers of various ailments. When facing a disease, you not only need courage and faith, but also belief in miracles.

December 30, 2004

Introduction
to Traditional Chinese Medicine

The Basic Principles

Traditional Chinese medicine (TCM) has its roots in the ancient philosophy of Taoism, which originated in China more than 3,000 years ago. The Taoists believed the universe to be an infinite web of complex and ever-changing patterns. The expression of these patterns is carried out by two opposing yet complementary primal forces, Yin and Yang, which we human beings perceive as a variety of opposing qualities, such as day and night, heat and cold, excess and deficiency, interior and exterior, activity and rest. The interactions between such opposing qualities weave the grand patterns of the universe. Everything in nature exhibits varying combinations of both Yin and Yang; nothing is purely one or the other and one has no meaning without the other. In the human body, just as in nature, a fine balance between Yin and Yang must be maintained for good health. When the balance is upset, illness or dysfunction occurs.

The view of Western medicine emphasizes the physical structures of the human body. Anatomy and physiology study these structures from the largest bones, muscles, and skin to the smallest cells or even molecules. This structural map forms the basis of modern medicine. In contrast, the traditional Chinese medicine model emphasizes process rather than structure. The human body is seen as an energy system in which various substances—such as *Qi*, *Blood*, *Jing*, *Body Fluids*, and *Shen*—interact with each other to create the whole physical organism. Among these substances, Qi is the most important. Qi is a vital essence that is part matter, part energy. Qi flows within a closed system of channels, or so-called meridians, throughout the human body. This network of meridians allows Qi to reach all the tissues and organs, providing nourishment, warmth, and energy to all parts of the body. If this flow is weakened or blocked in any way, the ensuing imbalance in turn will manifest itself as illness.

Western medicine relies on modern technologies—from stethoscope to MRI (magnetic resonance imaging)—to monitor patients' physical, chemical, and pathological statuses in order to make a diagnosis. Of course, during its thousands of years of development, TCM learned to utilize quite different techniques. They are *Looking*, *Listening and Smelling*, *Questioning and Touching*. Through these techniques the practitioner analyzes the information gathered and reaches a diagnosis. Instead of naming a specific disease, as is done in the Western medicine, the Chinese practitioner diagnoses what kinds of imbalances, such as a certain type of Yin deficiency or Yang excess, exist in the body. Then, the practitioner tailors an individual treatment plan according to these disharmonies.

Although the meridians are deep within the body, points along them are accessible from the surface of the skin. At such points, a traditional Chinese healer can manipulate the flow of Qi by pressure, heat, or needle, bringing healing essence to the organs that need it. In general, the goal of all TCM therapy is to regulate Qi and other substances to ensure their optimal flow and to keep the balance of Yin and Yang in the human body. Traditional Chinese medicine works totally different from Western medicine, because it does not treat the disease; rather it treats the whole person through harmonizing within.

How to Use TCM for Your Own Healthcare

Traditional Chinese medicine and Western medicine both have advantages and disadvantages. They often complement each other and alternate in their leading roles. One becomes the complementary medicine of the other, depending on the clinical condition of the patient, so integration of two medical systems is the key to your own health.

If you have any symptoms that concern you, see your physician first. Depending upon the diagnosis, you can choose which treatment is in your best interest. It could be only the Western approach, only Chinese medicine, or it could be a combination of both. After visiting your physician, you will know if you can treat yourself at home.

Another kind of integration involves all aspects of TCM— Chinese herbs, acupuncture, moxibustion, scraping, cupping, Chinese massage, reflexology, Tai Chi, and Qi Gong. Each of these therapies has its own advantages. They complement each other. If you combine these different therapies into your daily life over the long term, you will get excellent results for many chronic diseases.

Finally, be open-minded. Keeping a positive attitude is essential in getting the most from traditional Chinese medicine. Try not to interpret every detail of TCM with the language used by Western medicine. They are totally different systems. (*Note*: The Appendix includes a quick measurement conversion chart for use with the recipes and remedics included in each section.)

Part One

Self-Healing Approaches in Traditional Chinese Medicine

Traditional Chinese medicine uses many kinds of therapeutic methods. Here are brief descriptions of the therapies, which are convenient for self-application.

Chinese Herbs

The Chinese practice of using herbs to cure illness is believed to date back some 4,000 years. A very old Chinese legend says that in the remote past there lived a man named Shen Nong, or God of Husbandry, who tasted hundreds of kinds of herbs to determine their therapeutic values. Over a long period of time, the Chinese accumulated enormous experience and developed a unique pharmaceutical system, which has proven to be the best natural therapy for treating all kinds of illnesses.

Chinese "herbs" include not just plants, but also minerals and parts of animals. They are divided into five energy categories: cold, cool, hot, warm, and neutral. They have five taste qualities: sour/astringent, sweet, bitter, salty, and pungent/acrid. These tastes and energetic properties describe the therapeutic effects of the herbs.

Herbs can be used individually, but they are often used in combination with others, which is called a *formula*.

What Types of Chinese Herbs Can You Use?

- **Raw herbs.** The traditional way to take Chinese herbs is to drink a tea concocted from raw herbs according to the prescription, which is tailored to the patient's individual pattern of disharmony. Typically, they are provided in a bag that contains raw, dried roots, leaves, and seeds. At home, the patient cooks this mixture according to the practitioner's instructions and then drains off the resulting brew for drinking.

- **Herb tincture.** Sometimes an herb or a combination of herbs is soaked in water or alcohol, and sealed for a certain period of time to extract the effective constituents. This kind of herb is called a *tincture*.

- **Patent herbs.** Many of the classic formulas that have been developed over the centuries are considered so useful that they are manufactured in readily available patent form, such as herbal tablets, herbal honey balls, ointments, or patches and sprays.

- **Herb extract.** The extracts of herb products have become widely used in the last 10 years. Through a complex series of processing steps, the herbs are transformed into small granules that are easily measured and used.

What Else Do You Need to Know About Herbs?

- Herbs are not always harmless. Generally speaking, herbs are a kind of dietary supplement. Taking a little more or a little less will not affect the body much. But sometimes an overdose of any kind of herb has a negative effect. The patient needs to strictly follow the instructions indicated by the practitioner. In the United States, federal regulations categorize most of the Chinese herbs as dietary supplements, not as medicine.

- Some herbs are contraindicated during pregnancy. Read the description very carefully. If you have a serious heart problem, diabetes, or cancer, please consult with professionals.

Food Therapy

Yi Shi Tong Yuan is an ancient Chinese proverb that means "medicine and diet both originate from the practice and experience of daily life." The concept of proper diet as therapy has a very long tradition. In *The Yellow Emperor's Classic of Medicine*, which is the seminal text in TCM that was written 3,000 years ago, several medicated diet prescriptions were recorded. Since then TCM has accumulated a vast repository of knowledge about the therapeutic values of a great variety of food, which can include many kinds of cereals, fruits, nuts, vegetables, animals, and seafood. Therapeutic food can also be taken in combination with salutary herbs and condiments, an approach called *medicated diet*. In light of its form and process, medicated diet can be divided into five types:

- **Fresh Juice:** the juice extracted from edible Chinese herbs alone.
- **Herbal Tea:** the coarsely mixed powder of herbs with tea leaves that is to be taken frequently as ordinary tea dissolved in boiling water.
- **Medicated Wine:** a liquid dose made by combining wine with some kind of plant. It can be made either by infusing or brewing.
- **Medicated Soup:** the liquid prepared by combining specific vegetables, fruits, meats, rice, and water.
- **Cooked Dishes:** a large group of medicated diet recipes, including a variety of curative meat and vegetable dishes.

According to Chinese medicine, the natures of all foods fall into three different categories:

- *Hot or Warm:* ginger, walnuts, red dates, lamb, fennel, for example. This kind of food has the function of warming internally the body, dispelling cold, and restoring Yang. So they are used to treat illness with Yin and/or cold syndrome.
- *Cold or Cool Type:* mung beans, lotus, watermelon, water chestnuts, bitter melon, chrysanthemum, for example. This kind of food has the function of removing heat and clearing toxin, so they are used to treat illness with heat syndrome.

☙ *Neutral Type:* pork, beef, for example. This kind of food is moderate, neither too hot nor too cold, and is used with other types of food.

Besides the nature of the food, there are also five different tastes or flavors. They are sour, bitter, sweet, pungent, and salty. They have special meaning with regard to therapeutic effect. A correct food therapy must be based on the nature and taste of all ingredients, which can balance the syndrome of the illness.

What Else Do You Need to Know About Food Therapy?

☙ Chinese medicine emphasizes maintaining appropriate diet—what you should eat and what you shouldn't eat. There is a type of food called *overstimulating food*, which is a type of food that exacerbates existing symptoms or creates new symptoms when injested during the duration of the condition. For different conditions there are different overstimulating foods. What food is overstimulating depends on your constitution, genetic factors, seasonal effects and even emotions. For a person with internal heat, lamb is an overstimulating food, but lamb is the perfect choice for a person with internal cold. A person with asthma may eat whatever he/she likes, but, if an attack occurs, milk, fish, shrimp, and eggs can become overstimulating foods and may trigger a problem.

☙ Another category of food is called *incompatible food*, which reduces the therapeutic effects or brings up some side effects when you are taking one specific herb. For example, radish and ginseng can't be eaten together.

Chinese Massage (Tui Na)

Like other elements of TCM, Chinese massage, or Tui Na, has a long history and dates back to ancient times. It is a simple therapy that uses neither medicine nor medical devices, but only various massage techniques to stimulate the body to regulate bodily functions and eliminate harmful factors. Chinese massage can regulate and balance the Yin and Yang of the human body, and improve the functions of the meridians and the circulation of Qi and the blood.

Over thousands of years, Chinese massage has evolved into a successful, systematic healthcare method for treating a wide range of disorders, including those addressed by internal medicine, surgery, gynecology, pediatrics, and emergency rooms. Generally speaking, it is most helpful for chronic conditions.

Through time, Chinese massage has grown into many academic schools and branches. Among them, *acupressure* is one of the most commonly used variations because of its convenience and effectiveness. The unique nature of acupressure makes it accessible and affordable to everybody, so it is widely accepted by people around the world. The Japanese version of acupressure is known as *Shiatsu*.

Commonly Used Acupressure Techniques

Although TCM practitioners use a variety of acupressure techniques, here is a brief explanation of some of the main techniques you can use at home. When you do self-massage, it is not necessary to worry if the technique you use is not exactly the same as described in this book. Just use the one that feels best to you.

- **Pressing.** With the fingertip or the heel of the palm, or the tip of the joint of the fingers, continuously press the target area, varying the pressure from light to heavy, from shallow to deep.
- **Kneading.** With a fingertip or the heel of the palm, or the pad in the thumb's side of the palm, knead slowly and softly, back and forth or circularly, over the target region. The hand should remain fixed on the target area without any rubbing or slipping on the surface. But it should bring the underlying muscles to move.
- **Rubbing.** Using the palm or the palm side of the fingers, gently rub the target area in a circular motion.
- **Pushing.** Using the thumb or the palm, or the edge of the hand, scrape the target area along a straight line slowly in one direction only.
- **Scrubbing.** Using the palm or the edge of the hand, scrub the target area back and forth along a straight line. It is similar to pushing, but in both directions with less pressure.

- ☞ **Grasping.** With thumb and fingers, slowly lift and squeeze the target area.
- ☞ **Patting.** Using an open palm, pat and beat the surface of the body.
- ☞ **Rub rolling.** Using both palms, hold both sides of the target area. Simultaneously to rub and twist the target back and forth rapidly, move the palms up and down slowly in the target area. Do not skim the surface of the skin, but it should bring the underlying muscles to move. Most times it is used for the ribcage, shoulders, and limbs.
- ☞ **Wiping.** Using the surface of the thumb or fingers, softly and rhythmically rub the skin of the target area back or forth. Most times it is applied to the head.

Commonly Used Points

The human body has 14 channels and more than 300 points, each of which is sensitive and relevant to some particular illness. Each channel and point is assigned a scientific symbol. Locating these points is essential for getting the best results from Chinese massage. The bone-length measurement and finger-length measurement are used mostly by professional practitioners. At home, you can use the measurement according to the part of the body and your finger length. In self-treatment, it is not as critical to locate these points.

What Else Should You Know About Chinese Massage?

- ☞ Apply massage oil or talcum powder to lubricate and protect the skin. Trim your nails.
- ☞ As a home remedy, every application should be gentle. If it feels uncomfortable, application should be light and soft. If it still doesn't feel good, stop.
- ☞ Don't practice after strenuous exercise. Don't practice with a totally empty or full stomach. Don't practice if you are extremely weak or right after recovering from a severe disease.
- ☞ Massage does not treat severe heart disease, mental disorders, cancer, or acute infectious diseases.

- It should not be used on open wounds or any skin problems such as dermatitis, burns, bruises, and scalds.
- Do not massage a new injury that shows swelling, or if it is hot to touch.
- Massage can't be applied to the abdomen or the lower back of women with menses or who are pregnant.

Qi Gong (Mind Exercise)

Regulating your Qi is vital to your health. Although Qi can be manipulated by a practitioner or with herbs, it can also be harnessed by yourself to enhance your health. Qi Gong is a physical and meditative art designed to cultivate Qi. Through a combination of measured body movement and breathing control, one can focus Qi and facilitate its flow through the meridians. Simply put, Qi Gong is a long-term exercise of mind and breath control to regulate the whole body-energy-spirit system.

Qi Gong Practice

Start a Qi Gong practice session with some warm-up sequences. Rub your hands, massage your head and face, move and stretch the neck and shoulders, and so on. Most importantly, calm your mind down, let your spirit be at peace, and achieve a relaxed but concentrated focus on the exercise.

What follows depends on the protocols of specific Qi Gong disciplines. In general, you will take a certain posture and use different breath techniques to conduct the Qi in your body. The whole process of learning or practicing Qi Gong is about regulating the following three key elements:

- **Regulation of Body:** This refers to the adjustment of body postures and relaxation exercises. You need to relearn how to sit, stand, and move because the effectiveness of an exercise depends on the correct posture or movement. Ideally, a posture is natural and easy. It is not forced by willpower and tension, but sustained by Qi power.
  - *Lying:* You can lie on your back or on your side. This is the easiest way to relax the whole body.

▷ *Sitting:* If you sit on a chair, be sure that your feet rest fully on the ground. Place them parallel to each other, toes pointing to the front, shoulder width apart. Imagine your feet and the earth beneath them really belonging to each other. When you sit, the emphasis is on outer stillness and inner Qi movement.

▷ *Standing:* Stand with feet parallel, toes pointing to the front, about shoulder width apart; knees slightly bent. Your weight is distributed equally between both feet. Relax your knees. Your upper body is upright without being stiff, your chin slightly tucked. Eyes are half closed. Relax the neck. Imagine your head is in the heavens and your feet are rooted in the earth.

☞ **Regulation of Breathing:** This refers to the exercise of respiration and conducting Qi. There are two basic methods:

▷ *Natural Breathing*: the ordinary breathing pattern; good for a beginner.

▷ *Belly Breathing*: While inhaling, expand the abdomen. While exhaling, contract the abdomen. This breathing technique develops gradually with practice until it occurs naturally.

☞ **Regulation of Mind:** This refers to the regulation of mental activities including tranquilization and concentration. The following three methods are most common:

▷ *Mind Concentration*: Concentrate the mind on certain parts of the body, an acupuncture point, or an object outside the body. The concentration should be natural and unstrained, with no forced exertion.

▷ *Silent Reciting*: Silently recite a certain single word or phrase. For example, the words "relax" and "peace." One word for exhalation and another word for inhalation respectively. Its purpose is to replace the jumble of thoughts that clutter the mind with one pure thought, and to gradually achieve a state free from stray thoughts and full of relaxation, and joy, and tranquility.

▷ *Mental Imaging*: Use the mind's eye to look inward at a certain part inside your own body or outward at an object outside your body to induce a tranquil state of mind.

How much benefit you can gain from Qi Gong is dependent on how well you can master and coordinate these key elements.

Finish your exercise with some ending sequences. First conduct the Qi to the area two finger-widths below your bellybutton. Slowly open your eyes, take several deep breaths, stretch your legs, and take a two-minute rest.

What Else Do You Need to Know About Qi Gong?

- Like Chinese massage, Qi Gong has developed an immense variety of styles and forms. Some are very simple, and others are very complex. Some of them target health maintenance, and others emphasize self-defense.

- If you use Qi Gong to treat a particular illness, and you can't hold the specified posture, do your best to adjust your body so that it is in the most comfortable and relaxed state possible. Also, if you can't do belly breathing well, change it to natural breathing. However, if you do want to systematically master Qi Gong for long-term healthcare, you need to join a Qi Gong class.

- If saliva accumulates during the practice, swallow it three times. Never spit it out.

- If you feel tired during the practice, concentrate your mind on the area two finger-widths below your belly button for a while or change to normal breathing.

- Practice Qi Gong in the outdoors in a natural setting or in a quiet room filled with fresh air.

- Don't practice right after a meal. Don't practice when you are exhausted.

- Very rarely, a person can have a physical or mental (over) reaction from Qi Gong practice. This could come in the form of dizziness, shortness of breath, or uncontrolled movement of arms and legs. If this happens, don't panic. You can massage the areas where you feel uncomfortable, and take a good rest. You should stop the exercise and consult with experienced Qi Gong instructors.

Heat Therapy (Moxibustion)

In Chinese, the phrase "acupuncture" is composed of two words, *Zhen Ju*. *Zhen* means "needle," which is a well-known technique already familiar to the American public. *Ju* is "moxibustion," which is much less familiar.

Moxibustion is a type of heat therapy. By lighting a cigar-like moxa stick over the acupuncture point, the heat will penetrate into the meridians to regulate the Qi and blood in the same way as a needle. Moxibustion can treat almost every illness as well as acupuncture can. It can either be used as a complementary approach to other therapies, or as a stand-alone therapy.

In the West, practitioners only use indirect moxibustion, where the moxa is burned indirectly, either above the skin or on another medium between the moxa and the skin. For example, the medium can be sliced garlic, sliced ginger, or salt.

To keep things simple we use the term *heat therapy* in place of moxibustion. Also, we suggest you use moxa only above the skin, and be careful not to touch the burning stick to your skin or let the hot ashes of moxa burn you.

Folk Remedies

Folk remedy refers to simple herbal formulas (usually consisting of one or two herbs) or a technique that has specific therapeutic effects for one particular illness. Folk remedies have been circulating among ordinary people for ages and enjoy a great deal of popularity. The folk remedy is a part of traditional Chinese medicine.

Folk remedies may only work for certain conditions. Every person has a different constitution and becomes ill in different situations. A disease has Yin or Yang nature with either excess or deficiency. A syndrome may be hot or cold either exterior or interior. If you don't feel a remedy helps after several tries, stop using it.

Tai Chi Quan

If you have ever visited China or seen a documentary on the daily life in its cities, you probably have seen fascinating early morning scenes of elderly Chinese moving together in a slow, dance-like form in the neighborhood park. They are practicing *Tai Chi Quan* (or known simply as Tai Chi, or Tai Ji), a Chinese movement therapy. It was first devised by a Taoist monk in the 13th century. Literally translated, Tai Chi Quan means "supreme ultimate boxing art."

Tai Chi is the Dynamic Form of Qi Gong

Tai Chi and Qi Gong share a common philosophical background: they share the aim to harmonize the Yin and the Yang energies, and smooth Qi throughout the body. Tai Chi combines breathing techniques and sequences of movements to improve the flow of Qi, calm the mind, and promote self-healing. Its sequence is a slow series of postures, linked into one long, flowing exercise, which are designed to focus body and mind in harmony to encourage an even flow of Qi.

Tai Chi has many forms. The *empty hand form* is the most popular practice taught to all ages in the West.

Benefits of Practicing Tai Chi

Tai Chi is practiced more as a form of preventive healthcare than as a response to an ailment. It is becoming increasingly well known as a way of reducing stress and improving peace of mind and spiritual well-being. Beyond that, recent medical research has found that T'ai Chi practice will bring more energy, stabilize blood pressure, enhance the immune system, increase breathing capacity, and improve posture control. For the elderly, it makes them less likely to injure themselves by falling.

In this book, Tai Chi will be mentioned on many occasions. If you are interested in learning how to practice, there are many Tai Chi classes available in most communities, and books and instructional videos are also readily available.

Part Two

Self-Healing With
Traditional Chinese Medicine
Home Remedies from A to Z

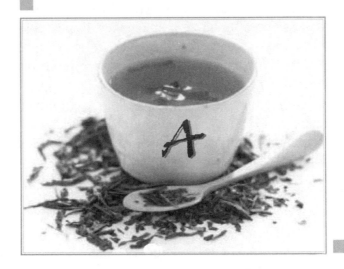

Acne

WHAT IS IT AND WHAT CAUSES IT?

It can be pimples, whiteheads, red blemishes, and skin cysts on your face or body (especially chest and back). Most of the time acne occurs in youth. In adolescence, acne is related to hormonal changes. Oil glands secrete too much sebum, which clogs the pores. Also genetics, stress, cosmetics, and some medications can cause the problem.

WHEN SHOULD YOU SEE A DOCTOR?

If your skin is inflamed with cysts or nodules, or there is no response to your self-treatment, see a doctor.

WHAT SHOULD YOU DO IN DAILY LIFE?

- If the acne is not broken yet, wash your face with warm or hot water and baby soap two times a day.
  - Make soap bubbles with warm water as much as possible in a basin. Use both hands to wash your face with these soap bubbles for one minute.

- Use hot water from a shower (as hot as you feel comfortable) to rinse your face for 20 seconds. Meanwhile use your palm gently to pat your face. Then use warm water to rinse for another 20 seconds. Repeat this cycle three times.
- Using a towel, gently press your face to absorb the water.

- Keep your diet free of greasy, spicy, fatty, and fried foods. Chinese medicine thinks those kinds of foods cause internal heat or damp toxin, which lead to acne. Eat more vegetables such as raw cucumbers, bitter melon, mushrooms, diakon radish, winter melons, celery, tomatoes, tofu, lotus, watermelon, and pears to get rid of heat in the body.
- Acne may be caused by an allergic reaction to certain food such as milk, eggs, pineapple, bananas, or mangoes. Try to find out if this is the case for you.
- Have regular bowel movements and avoid constipation.
- Get plenty of sleep. The metabolic process that removes excess oil from your skin works best between 10 p.m. and 2 a.m. during sleep.

WHAT SHOULDN'T YOU DO?

- Don't pick at your face or squeeze the pimples.
- If possible, don't wear makeup. Otherwise, only use water-based makeup and remove all cosmetics before bedtime.
- If sweating a lot, don't immediately wash your face with cold water or walk into a room with an air conditioner.
- Avoid alcohol and smoking. Don't eat desserts with a lot of sugar or cream. Try to cut out dairy products. These all can cause acne or make it worse.
- Avoid emotional upsets and get plenty of rest to reduce stress and tension.

Folk Remedies

- Wash your face with warm water mixed with three drops of honey every evening. Gently massage pimples for five minutes. Let the skin absorb the honey. Wash again with clear, warm water.

- Apply one of the following options as mask. Do a skin test first. If you have an allergic reaction, stop using the mask.

  - Grind 1/2 oz. orange seeds (available in Chinese herb stores). Mix with an egg white to make a paste. Apply for 40 minutes. Wash mask off.

  - Smash a ripe tomato. Add 1 tsp. of oak powder and make a paste. Apply to the pimples. Wash off when the mask is dry.

  - Grind several Vitamin B6 tablets. Mix Vitamin B6 powder with water to make a paste. Apply to the acne for 40 minutes, once a day.

  - Slice fresh aloe vera. Use it to rub and knead the acne twice a day. If you have an allergic reaction stop using the mask. You can also try lemon instead of aloe vera.

Food Therapy

- Drink pearl barley soup:

  Ingredients: 2 oz. Chinese pearl barley, 1 tsp. sugar.

  Procedure: Add 3 cups of water to ingredients to make barley soup. Make and drink one batch a day for two weeks.

- Drink vegetable juice:

  Ingredients: 3 oz. celery, 1 tomato, 1 Asian pear, 1/4 lemon.

  Procedure: Remove the center from the pear. Put the rest of the pear and other ingredients in a juicer. Make and drink this juice once a day for two weeks.

- Eat mung bean and lily soup:

Ingredients: 1 oz. mung beans, 1 oz. lily bulb (available in Chinese grocery stores), 1/4 oz. sugar.

Procedure: Soak the mung beans in water overnight. Add 3 cups of water and bring to a boil. Reduce heat and simmer until beans are soft. Add sugar for flavor and drink once a day for two weeks.

Chinese Massage

☞ Dry wash your face: Sitting with your eyes closed, rub two hands against each other until they are warm. Use four fingers to wipe your face from your forehead downward, to the lips, to the lower jaw, to underneath the ears, then circle back, upward to the temples. Do this 10 times, then repeat in the opposite direction.

☞ Choose the following and massage each point for one minute once a day.

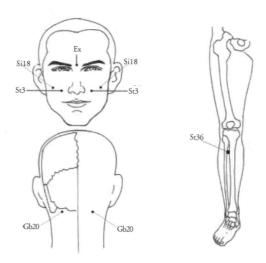

☞ Gently press and knead the point located above the bridge of your nose halfway between the inner edges of each eyebrow (Ex).

- ☛ Gently press and knead the points on the cheek directly under the eye pupil and level with the low edge of the nostril (St3).
- ☛ Gently press and knead the points under the cheekbone in line with the outer corner of the eye (Si18).
- ☛ Gently press and knead the point in the depression at the bottom of the skull, outside of the two big muscles on the neck, which you can feel by bending your neck forward, head down (Gb20).
- ☛ Gently press and knead the depression that is four finger-widths below the kneecap edge and one thumb-width outside of the shinbone (St36).

Chinese Herbs

- ☞ Use the patented herb Acne Getaway 101E. Follow the instructions.

Addiction

WHAT IS IT?

A bodily dependency on a substance of a bad habit such as nicotine or alcohol.

WHAT SHOULD YOU DO?

- ☞ When you decide to quit your habit, if you feel you are strong enough, you can just stop the cigarettes or alcohol right away. Otherwise, you may go slowly to cut down the amount gradually.
- ☞ Tell your family and friends that you are quitting your bad habit. Let people keep an eye on you.
- ☞ You should first stay away from everything related to your bad habit.
- ☞ Keep yourself busy so your mind won't stray to thoughts of temptation.
- ☞ Practice Tai Chi. Let your mind follow the movement of your hands—let your mind follow your Qi (vital energy).

WHAT SHOULDN'T YOU DO?

- Don't keep cigarettes or liquor at home. Don't go to a bar before you can control yourself.
- Refrain from talking to people when they are smoking or accompanying people on their cigarette breaks.

Folk Remedies

- Prepare a small piece of ginseng. When you are getting an urge to smoke, keep the ginseng between your lips and suck on it, telling yourself that this is good for your health. This may give you a sense of contentment.
- If you have an urge to have a cigarette, slowly sip a cup of warm water.

Food Therapy

- Eat radish to quit smoking: Shred 2 oz. of diakon radish into small pieces. Squeeze the excessive juice. Mix in 1 tsp. of sugar and let stand overnight. Eat them in the morning.
- Eat tofu with sugar to quit smoking: Get half box of tofu. Punch several holes in tofu and fill in with some brown sugar. Steam them until well done. Take 3 Tbs. when you have an urge to have a cigarette.
- Drink black sesame seed, mulberry, and rice soup to quit alcohol:

    Ingredients: 1 oz. black sesame seeds, 1 oz. mulberry, 1/4 oz. sugar, 1 oz. rice

    Procedure: Grind sesame seeds, mulberry, and rice into a fine powder. Add 2 cups of water and bring to boil. Reduce heat and simmer for 20 minutes. Add sugar and divide into two portions. Eat twice daily.

Chinese Massage

When an urge strikes, use index fingers to massage your ears. First, start with the front area of ears, then the behind of ears, finally the interior folds. Repeat until the urge subsides.

Chinese Herbs

☞ Take zizyphus jujube granule, which is the kernel of a kind of wild date. Take 1 tsp. mixed with 1 cup of warm water and sip slowly three times a day. It relieves the anxiety of cigarette cravings. If you are trying to quit alcohol, take 1 tsp. of the powder three times a day or whenever the craving starts.

☞ Take pueraria root to quit alcohol. Mix 2 oz. of pueraria root powder with 1 cup of water. Simmer it on low heat to make a paste. Divide the paste into three portions. Take it three times a day.

☞ Drink herb tea to quit alcohol:

Ingredients: 1/8 oz. hawthorn fruit, 1/8 oz. chrysanthemum flower, 1/8 oz. honeysuckle flower.

Procedure: Add boiling water and cover with lid to steep for five minutes. Drink as tea.

Age Spots

WHAT IS IT AND WHAT CAUSES IT?

They are flat, freckle-like patches that mostly show up on your face and back of your hands. They may be caused by too much exposure to sunlight and poor liver function.

WHEN SHOULD YOU CALL A DOCTOR?

To avoid skin cancer, if the freckle-like patches change size or color, see a doctor.

WHAT SHOULD YOU DO IN DAILY LIFE?

- Wear a hat when outside. The hat should have a large brim to shield your face against the UV rays.
- Eat more vegetables and fruits, particularly onion. When cooking, use vegetable oil only.
- Drink plenty of water daily.
- Exercise regularly.

WHAT SHOULDN'T YOU DO?

- Reduce the intake of fat in your diet.

Folk Remedies

- Take rice vinegar: Every morning on an empty stomach, drink a mixture of 1 Tbs. of vinegar and 1 Tbs. of honey in 1 oz. of warm water.
- Cut lemon into very small chunks and rub the spots three times a day. The acid in the lemon can remove the superficial layer of skin.
- Apply aloe vera gel twice a day.
- Break a Vitamin E soft gel and apply it on your age spots once a day.

Food Therapy

- Eat white fungus with quail egg:

  Ingredients: 1 oz. Chinese white fungus, 1 quail egg, 30 ml Chinese cooking wine.

  Procedure: Soak white fungus in water for three hours. Boil the eggs until well done and peel. Place all ingredients in a pot with 1/2 cup water. Use low heat to simmer until they are very soft. Add salt and eat one batch once a day for two weeks.

- Drink ginger with honey:

Ingredients: 3 slices ginger, 1 tsp. honey.

Procedure: Shed ginger into thin pieces. Steep in boiled water for 10 minutes. Add honey. Drink once a day for three weeks.

Chinese Massage

☞ Pat the back of your hand: Use your right palm to gently pat the back of your left hand until it is slightly red. Change hands to pat the other hand. Do it twice a day for a prolonged period.

☞ Rub your palms against each other until they are warmand then rub the affected areas, massaging the afdfected areas until you feel warm. Do this twice a day.

Chinese Herbs

☞ Drink fleece flower root tea.

Ingredients: 1/2 oz. processed fleece flower root, water.

Procedure: Cut the fleece flower root into small pieces. Soak them in a coffee maker with boiled water for four to eight hours until the color becomes brownish red. Drink it as tea. When the water is depleted, add more boiled water into the coffee maker to continue drinking, until the color of the tea becomes lighter. Drink for a month.

Anxiety

WHAT IS IT AND WHAT CAUSES IT?

Anxiety encompasses a broad field of emotional disorders such as panic attacks and phobias. Experts believe both underlying biological and psychological issues can cause the problem. The symptoms are insomnia, excessive tension, and nervousness. Here we will focus on treatments targeting the psychological roots, such as prolonged periods of stress.

WHEN SHOULD YOU CALL A DOCTOR?

If you experience persistent anxiety, or if you feel the symptoms are changing your life, see a doctor.

WHAT SHOULD YOU DO IN DAILY LIFE?

- Exercise regularly, such as practicing Tai Chi.
- Eat calcium-rich and amino acid-rich foods such as milk, bean products, fish, shrimp, chicken, beef, bananas, or dates. Calcium and amino acid can help to calm you down.
- Be sure to sleep well.

WHAT SHOULDN'T YOU DO?

- Do not suppress or hide your worries and fears. Talk to family members or friends you can trust about your worries and the injustices you have suffered. Emotional release is a good, natural necessity in mental health. When you share them, the toxicity disappears.
- Don't eat spicy food such as onions, ginger, and peppers. In Chinese medical theory, anxiety is caused by internal fire. The spicy food could ignite the fire.

Folk Remedies

- When you are experiencing anxiousness, use "aroma therapy."
  - Put freshly peeled skins of your favorite fruit in a bottle with a big opening. Breathe slowly and deeply into the bottle.
  - Buy enough dried white chrysanthemum from a Chinese herb store to fill a 4 x 6-inch cotton fabric bag. Breathe slowly and deeply into the bag. Use bag until the aroma disappears.
  - Rub two drops of lavender oil on the hair above your forehead. The aroma of lavender oil has calming effects on the nervous system.
- Use a wood comb gently to brush your head (hair) from the forehead to the back of your head, from the center to both sides. Use adequate force. Do this for three minutes once a day. The tip of the comb should not be sharp.
- Treating your feet can moderate your autonomic nerve, which plays a very important role in your anxiety.
  - Soak your feet in hot water (as hot as you feel comfortable) for 20 minutes every day. If the water reaches

your calf, you can get a better result. After soaking, rotate your ankles 20 times, one after another. Use your hand to rotate each toe clockwise 20 times, then counter clockwise 20 times. Meanwhile repeatedly, silently talk to yourself "calm down, calm down."

- ☞ Use a soft brush to brush your soles for five minutes. Pay special attention to the point below the ball of the foot in the center, about a third of the distance between the toes and the heel. Before brushing, apply some cream to protect your skin.

- ☞ Use an empty plastic soft drink bottle to pat your bare foot (the top, the sole, and both sides) for three minutes. Keep your knock rhythmically about three times per second. Tap each location about 30 times.

☞ Massage your ears: Sit on a chair. Use the thumb and the outside of the index finger to grab your ear and pull in different directions (upwards, downwards, horizontally) for 30 seconds. Grab another location and repeat the same procedure. Meanwhile deeply and slowly inhale and exhale.

Qi Gong

☞ In the evening when the moon has just risen, stand facing the moon in a quiet backyard. Place your feet shoulder width apart. Raise your hands to the moon with the palms up, as to hug the moon. Place your tongue against the palate. Breath naturally. Inhale and visualize the essence of the moon coming down to your palms. Place one hand on the top of the head. Overlap with the other palm. Close your eyes. Imagine the essence of the moon pouring into your body from the vertex. Exhale. Repeat this five times. In Chinese medicine the sun is Yang and the moon is Yin. Anxiety is the imbalance of Yin and Yang with hyperactivity of Yang. The Yin essence of the moon will help the balance in your body.

☞ River of harmonious spirit:
  - ☞ Lie down comfortably in a quiet room, and take several deep breaths. Close your eyes and breathe naturally.

- ☞ Say to yourself "My head is relaxed, my face is relaxed, my neck is relaxed, my shoulders are relaxed, my arms are relaxed, my hands are relaxed, my fingers are relaxed, my chest is relaxed, my abdomen is relaxed, my legs are relaxed, my feet are relaxed, my toes are relaxed, my whole body is totally relaxed."

- ☞ Imagine a river flowing from the top center of your head down to your chest, stomach, and abdomen. Then the river divides into two streams that flow into each leg and come out from the soles of your feet. It flows away from you, flows on, becomes smaller and smaller, and finally disappears. Meanwhile, think of your worries and fear flowing along with this river, leaving you forever. Repeat this visualization once a day.

Chinese Massage

See **Depression** section.

Chinese Herbs

- ☞ Take the patent herb Dan Zhi Xiao Yao Wan. Follow the instructions.

Arthritis

WHAT IS IT AND WHAT CAUSES IT?

It is a general term for inflammation of the joints resulting in pain, stiffness and swelling in joints. It is a symptom of various diseases. Here we only introduce two kinds of the most common arthritis.

- ✽ **Osteoarthritis:** an age-related degeneration of cartilage in the joints.
- ✽ **Rheumatoid arthritis:** inflammation of the synovial membrane, which consists of lubricating fluid that protects the joints.

WHEN SHOULD YOU SEE A DOCTOR?

If you have newly developed joint stiffness, swelling, or redness, see your doctor for a diagnosis.

WHAT SHOULD YOU DO IN DAILY LIFE?

* Eating a well-balanced diet and drinking enough water are essential. Eat more foods rich in omega-3 fatty acids such as salmon, tuna, and sardines. From a Chinese medicine point of view, you need to eat more foods with tendons such as beef, chicken wing, or pig's feet.
* Exercise regularly: swimming, walking, dancing, and practicing Tai Chi.
* Take enough Vitamin C, D, E, omega-3s, fish oil, glucosamine and chondroitin sulfate for osteoarthritis.
* Control your weight.
* Take a mud bath, sand bath, or have hydrotherapy.

WHAT SHOULDN'T YOU DO?

* Avoid exposure to cold and damp conditions. Never sleep directly on the ground or sit on a rock for a long time. Avoid getting caught in the rain. If you do get caught, change your clothes immediately. Keep your home warm and dry.
* Avoid fatty or fried food. Avoid alcohol. Do not eat cold, raw food. Eat fewer lemons and oranges. Don't eat too many sweets.

Folk Remedies

* Wearing polyester underwear may provide some relief for joint pain, because of the static electricity effect.
* If your joint is not red and swollen, steam with vinegar:

  Ingredients: 300 ml rice vinegar, half a brick.

  Procedure: Place the brick in an oven or fireplace to warm it until it becomes hot. Dip a piece of gauze in vinegar and wrap it on the affected joint. Soak the brick in vinegar and place it about one foot beneath your joint. Steam for five minutes. Move your joint closer to the brick according to its temperature. Be careful with the hot brick.

🌾 If your joint is not red and swollen, apply fennel with salt:

Ingredients: 2 oz. fennel fruit, 8 oz. salt.

Procedure: Stir-fry fennel and salt in a pan until very hot. Wrap them in a cotton-based fabric. Apply the fennel and salt pack to the painful spot for one hour, twice a day for five days. Make a new pack for each application. Be careful with the heated salt.

🌾 If your joint is not red and swollen, apply cooked rice and salt:

Ingredients: 4 portions cooked rice, 1 portion salt.

Procedure: Mix rice with salt well. Place ingredients in a bowl and steam for two or three minutes. Wait until the temperature cools down to the point your skin feels comfortably warm. Wrap ingredients with cotton-based fabric. Apply it to the affected joint for one hour. Reheat if necessary. Do it once a day for five days.

🌾 If your joint is not red and swollen, apply ginger: Place 1 oz. of ginger into a juicer. Add to 1/2 cup of hot water to make ginger juice. Dip a piece of gauze in it and squeeze to dry. Apply to your painful spot. Repeat it two or three times a day. If you have an allergic reaction stop.

🌾 If your joint is not red and swollen, rub vinegar with green onion:

Ingredients: 500 ml rice vinegar, 1 lb green onion.

Procedure: Slice green onion into 1-inch long pieces and place in a pot with vinegar. Bring to a boil. Wait until as hot as you feel comfortable. Dip with gauze to rub and wash the painful spots for 10 to 30 minutes. Reheat vinegar if necessary. Do a skin test first, if you have an allergic reaction, discontinue use.

Food Therapy

🌾 If your joint is red and swollen, eat more tofu, pears, and mung beans. But do not eat pepper, cinnamon, ginger, or wine.

- ❧ If you have a painful and cold joint and an aversion to cold, eat lamb, ginger, papaya, or herb wine. Do not eat watermelon, kelp, pears, or mung beans.
- ❧ If you have a deformed joint and atrophic muscles, eat more chicken, neck bones, turtle, walnuts, or black sesame seeds.

Chinese Massage

Choose any combination of the following you feel comfortable with and do it once a day. If your joint is still hot and swollen, don't massage it.

- ❧ Gently press, knead, rub, and pat your painful spot for two minutes. According to the location of the pain, choose corresponding points to massage.

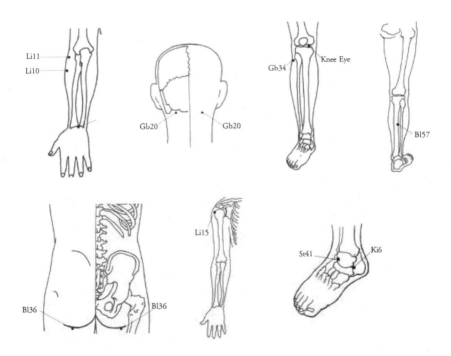

- ❧ If your finger or wrist is in pain, gently press and knead the point right in the depression where the wrist line meets the line from the ring finger, when the wrist is flexed slightly upward, for two minutes (Te4). Use your index finger to gently press the point on the forearm that is two thumb-widths below the crease of the elbow, in line with the thumb, for two minutes (Li10).

- If your elbow is in pain, gently press and knead Li10 (as previously) and the point at the end of the crease on the top of the elbow joint, with the arm folded across the chest, for two minutes (Li11).

- If your ankle is in pain, use your thumb to gently press the point in the middle of the front ankle crease, level with the anklebone, for two minutes (St41). Gently press the point on the inside of the ankle, one thumb-width below the tip of the anklebone, for two minutes (Ki6).

- If your knee is in pain, use your thumb to gently press the point on the outside of the leg, under the kneecap edge in the depression below the two lower leg bones' meeting point (Gb34). Gently press and knead both dents right below the kneecap at the inner and outside of the ligament with the knee bent for two minutes. Use both palms to rub the knee joint until it becomes warm.

- If your shoulders are in pain, knead and grasp the point on the top of the shoulder in the front depression (formed when you raise your arm parallel to the ground) for two minutes (Li15). Gently press and knead the point in the depression at the bottom of the skull, outside of the two big muscles on the neck, which you can feel by bending your neck forward, for two minutes (Gb20).

- If your hip joint is in pain, ask someone else to gently press and knead the back of the leg from the midpoint of the crease right below the buttock of the painful side (Bl36) down to the middle of the calf for two minutes (Bl57).

Chinese Herbs

- Take the patent herb Du Huo Ji Sheng Wan. Follow the instructions.

☞ If your joint is not red and swollen, apply a heating patch with herb, called Chinese Moxibustion. Follow the instructions.

Asthma

WHAT IS IT AND WHAT CAUSES IT?

It is a chronic lung disease that occurs when the bronchial tubes, which bring air into your lungs, become inflamed. Typical symptoms are shortness of breath, wheezing, coughing with phlegm, a suffocated feeling, and tightness in the chest.

Most asthma attacks are an over-reactive response to certain external triggers such as pollen, chemical, mold, smoke, viral respiratory infections, and activity. Asthma can also be caused by intrinsic conditions such as bronchitis or stressful emotion.

WHEN SHOULD YOU SEE A DOCTOR?

If you have any kind of breathing problem for the first time, or you are taking prescription medication for asthma but the symptoms are getting worse, see a doctor.

WHAT SHOULD YOU DO IN DAILY LIFE?

* Keep a diary to find the triggers and then avoid them.
* Drink coffee or warm water, which may widen your air channel.
* Eat Vitamin C-rich and calcium-rich food such as pumpkin, dates, oranges, tomatoes, green peppers, and tofu. From Chinese medicine's point of view, eat lotus seeds, chestnuts, Chinese yam, black beans, walnuts, pears, lily bulb, lamb, and Chinese white fungus.
* Control your emotions. Research shows 30 percent of asthma is caused by psychological factors such as anger, depression, or anxiety.
* Exercising every day is very important. Swimming is the best exercise for asthma. Qi Gong can make bronchus more relaxed. Walking one mile a day is good for your

heart and lungs. Take 20 minutes to walk a half mile first. Rest five minutes. Then walk another 20 minutes back to your home. Gradually increase the distance.

* Singing can help to relieve asthma because you have to use abdominal breathing instead of thoracic breathing. Abdominal breathing can increase vital capacity and reduce the pressure of lung.

* Beginning in the summer, use cold water to wash your face. Gradually advance to taking a short cold shower, if you can.

* If the doctor prescribed an inhaler for you, keep it with you all the time.

WHAT SHOULDN'T YOU DO?

* Do not smoke or drink alcohol.

* Reduce intake of salty food. Eliminate shrimp, crab, clams, and fish. For some people, seafood triggers an attack.

Folk Remedies

* Garlic helps you to fight asthma:
    * **Eat garlic with sugar:** Peel 1 lb. of garlic. Place bulbs in a pot with 1/2 lb. of crystal sugar. Add water to cover all. Bring to a boil and simmer until it looks like thick soup. Store in a jar. Drink 1 Tbs. twice a day. Stop if the garlic makes your stomach uncomfortable.
    * **Smell garlic:** Pound two cloves of garlic to paste and store in a small bottle. Smell it three times a day. Change the garlic every day.

Food Therapy

* Eat sugar with vinegar:

    Ingredients: 1 lb. sugar, 500 ml rice vinegar.

    Procedure: Place the sugar in a pot, add vinegar, and boil until sugar is dissolved. Store in a bottle. Take 10 ml two times a day. Follow by brushing your teeth.

- Eat pear with brown sugar: Remove the center of the pear and fill in with brown sugar. Steam until the sugar becomes sticky. Eat all while still warm.

- Take egg with green tea:

  Ingredients: 1/2 oz. green tea leaves, 2 eggs.

  Procedure: Place whole eggs and tea leaves in a pot with 2 cups of water. Cook until egg is well done. Peel shell off. Return eggs back to pot and continue to cook on low heat until all water is gone. Eat one egg a day.

- Eat black sesame seeds and walnuts with honey:

  Ingredients: 3 oz. black sesame seeds, 8 oz. walnuts, 100 ml honey.

  Procedure: Stir-fry walnuts and sesame seeds lightly on low heat. Smash walnuts into small pieces. Put walnuts, sesame seeds, and honey into a bowl with one cup of water. Stir well. Steam for 20 minutes. Eat 1 Tbs. at a time twice a day.

Chinese Massage

Choose the following and massage once a day:

- Use one thumb to gently press and knead the point on the pad of the thumb two finger-widths from the wrist, on the borderline between the dark and light skin, until you have a sensation of soreness and distention (Lu10). Change hands to do other side.

- Use your middle finger to gently press the dip between the collarbones above the breastbone for two minutes (Cv22). Meanwhile, use another middle finger to gently press the point right in the middle of the nipples for men, and between fourth and fifth ribs on the midline for women (Cv17).

- Use your middle fingers to gently press and knead the points on either side of the big bone at the base of the neck on the back for two minutes (Asthma point).

- If you have a lot of phlegm, gently press and knead the point on the outside edge of the leg bone, halfway between the tip of the anklebone and the middle of the knee-

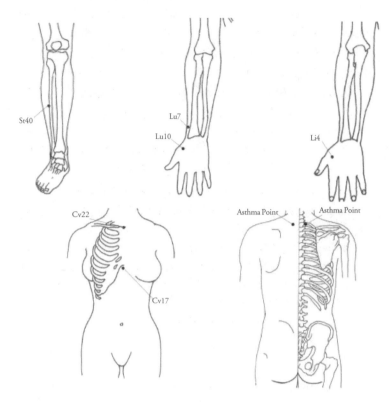

cap for one minute (St40).

☞ If you feel suffocated and short of breath, gently press the point right in the middle between the nipples for men, and between fourth and fifth ribs on the midline for women (Cv17). Do this for one minute.

☞ With your thumb against the index finger, use your other thumb to gently press the webbing where it bulges up the highest for one minute (Li4).

☞ Gently press the point located two finger-widths up from the wrist crease, on the inside of the forearm, in line with the thumb for one minute (Lu7).

☞ Use your thumb and fingers to gently, rhythmically, slowly grasp and release the front muscles of the neck along the trachea for one minute.

Qi Gong

☞ Stand in a quiet room, relax, and breathe naturally. Tap the upper and lower teeth together 36 times, stir the saliva inside the mouth with the tongue, and swallow the saliva.

☞ Imagine warm white air flowing into your lungs as you inhale deeply. Send the air slowly through the lungs down to the area two finger-widths below the belly button. Repeat this nine times.

☞ Place both palms on your chest. Inhale slowly. When you exhale, pronounce "sch." Meanwhile rub your chest with both palms from top to bottom. Repeat this six times.

☞ Sit on the ground with the legs naturally crossed. With your hands, press the ground on either side of your body, throw out your chest to inhale, pause awhile, then arc your back forward and draw in the chest to exhale. Repeat this six times.

☞ Sit in the lotus position. Place your palms on the knees. First twist to the left four times, then twist to the right four times. Inhale when you are turning to the left or right; exhale when you turn back.

Chinese Herbs

☞ Take 1/8 oz. of earthworm powder at a time, twice a day.

☞ Take herb with honey:

Ingredients: 1/4 oz. tendrilled fritillary bulb, 15 ml honey.

Procedure: Smash herb into small pieces. Add 2 cups of water and herbs to pot and cook for 30 minutes on low heat. Mix the decoction with honey. Drink once a day.

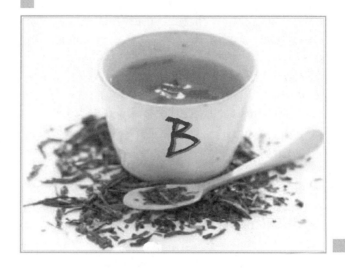

Back Pain (Chronic)

WHAT IS IT AND WHAT CAUSES IT?

Chronic back pain is persistent pain or stiffness in the lower back and waist. It may be caused by a disorder of the spine or the muscles in the back, such as arthritis, strain and sprain, muscle spasm, bone spur, or a herniated disk.

WHEN SHOULD YOU SEE A DOCTOR?

If you have a back pain, visit your doctor for a diagnosis to rule out other underlying diseases. If you have severe pain, or if it does not get better in two days, see your doctor.

WHAT SHOULD YOU DO IN DAILY LIFE?

- ⁎ In *acute* cases, resting is the first choice. Use ice in a plastic bag or a bag of frozen peas wrapped with a cloth to soothe the sore and inflamed area for 15 to 20 minutes. Repeat three to four times a day. (Acute cases usually only last a few days.)

- After one or two days, if the severe pain subsides, then you can use a heating pad with a warm, wet towel underneath for 20 minutes three to four times a day. You could use the heating pad three times, then an ice bag once daily. Repeat this cycle if necessary.

- Sleep on a bed with a firm mattress. Choose a comfortable pillow to keep your neck and spine in a natural position. If you lie on your side, put a pillow between your legs.

- In *chronic* cases, doing some of the following exercises regularly may help you relieve your back pain:

  - Walk forward in an S line for 10 minutes. Walk to the right for three or four steps, then to the left for three or four steps.

  - Walk like a penguin for five minutes. Keep your feet about 2 inches apart (toe turned out). Stand up naturally. Relax your knees. Slightly shake your body. Open your mouth and quietly pronounce "ah, ah." Slowly move forward. Don't lift your foot more than 1 inch.

  - Lie down on a hard floor. Pull both your knees toward your chest and lock both hands on the knees. Slowly rock your body back and forth to stretch your back for one or two minutes.

- Take some measures to protect your back in daily life:

  - Keep your back warm. Wear lumbar support if you have a weak back.

  - Wear comfortable shoes. Move your toes as much as possible, particularly the second toe. Walking barefoot at home, massaging your toes in the bath, and wearing slippers as much as possible can relieve and prevent back pain.

  - When lifting any heavy object, do some back exercises first. Hold the object close to your body and lift slowly.

  - If you work at a desk for prolonged time, adjust the height of your desk and chair properly. Change your body position or do some back exercise, every 30 minutes.

Place a small stool or box under your desk. Place your feet on it to raise your knee joint higher than the pelvic joint. In this way your sciatic nerve has less pressure and your spine is bending less.

✦ If you are going to drive for a prolonged time, be sure to use a backrest. If you don't have one, use a bath towel to support your back. Placing cardboard on the seat can also help.

✦ If you play golf, swing the club in the opposite direction several times before you prepare to hit a ball.

WHAT SHOULDN'T YOU DO?

⋈ When the back is in pain, avoid the activities that use the painful spot too much. It is not the right time to do exercise yet.

⋈ Don't sleep on damp ground or sit on a wet chair outdoors.

⋈ Don't bend your back directly to pick up things on the floor. Instead, bend your knees, then squat down and pick them up using your leg strength.

⋈ Don't wear high heel shoes, which may cause back pain for many women.

⋈ From Chinese medicine's point of view, don't have too much sex.

Folk Remedies

The following therapies are used in chronic cases only:

☞ Brush your feet, legs, and back for five to 10 minutes after a warm bath. Use a soft brush. The brush acts as a bunch of acupuncture needles. They stimulate the meridian and prompt the circulation of Qi and blood.

☞ Brush the soles and both sides of both feet, from the heel to the toes. Pay more attention to the point below the ball of the foot in the center, about a third of the distance between the toes and the heel. Before brushing, apply some cream to protect your skin.

⮞ Brush each toe from the root to the tip.

⮞ Brush the back of your leg, from the lower part of your calf, up to the back of your thigh.

⮞ Brush your back from the upper part down to the lower part.

❧ Blow the pain away: Set a hair dryer to low. Use it to blow warm air to the outside area under the kneecap to halfway down the leg. You can also blow warm air on the sole of your foot. If you feel too hot, move the hair dryer away a bit. When you feel the muscles cool down, move the hair dryer a bit closer. Take care not to burn yourself.

❧ Iron the pain away: Use three or four layers of cotton fabric to cover your back. Turn on a low-power iron for one minute, then **pull out the power line**. Ask a family member to slowly move the iron on the cotton fabric on your back, back and forth, just like ironing your clothes. Before ironing your back, make sure the temperature is warm, not hot. Take great care not to burn yourself.

❧ Steam several washcloths for 20 minutes. Wait until the cloth is comfortably hot to your skin. Apply to the painful spot. Cover the washcloth with clear plastic wrap for 15 minutes, after making sure the cloth is not too hot.

❧ Massage with a low-power vacuum cleaner: Sit on a chair. Take out the head or the brush of the vacuum cleaner. Use the opening of the pipe to gently suck at your back. Try to slightly lift the pipe, but don't lose contact with the skin. Continue for 10 seconds with suction while moving your back to the left, to the right, forward, or backward. Repeat several times.

❧ Hold your hands with fingers interlaced. Use your index and ring fingertips to gently press the points called "back pain points" (see the illustration on page 62), right underneath the tips 50 times. Meanwhile slowly rotate your back forward, backward, left, and right for two minutes. Do this whenever you have time.

☞ Apply hot salt on your back: Stir-fry 1 cup of salt in a pan until you can hear a cracking sound. Wrap the salt in a couple of paper towels, then with a cloth. Wait until the temperature cools down to the point of being comfortably hot on the skin. Apply to your back for one hour. Reheat if necessary.

☞ Wash with vinegar: Bring 300 ml rice vinegar to a boil. Wait until it cools to the point of being comfortably hot on your skin. Wash your painful spot for 15 minutes, once a day. Don't scald yourself. If you have an allergic reaction, discontinue use.

Food Therapy

☞ Drink spinach juice:

> **Ingredients:** 1 lb. spinach, Chinese cooking wine.
>
> **Procedure:** Make spinach juice with a juicer. Drink 100 ml of this juice with 30 ml wine, twice a day.

☞ Eat walnuts regularly:

> **Ingredients:** 7 walnuts shelled, 2 Tbs. brown sugar.
>
> **Procedure:** Stir-fry walnuts on low heat until a bit dark. Smash to small pieces and divide into two portions. Eat one portion with brown sugar, twice a day.

☞ Drink fruit wine:

> **Ingredients:** 7 figs, 500 ml 80-proof vodka.
>
> **Procedure:** Slice the figs into small strips. Soak them in vodka in a sealed bottle for seven days. Drink 25 ml at a time, twice a day for five days.

Chinese Massage

Choose from the following and massage once a day. In some cases, if you can't do it yourself, ask a family member to help you and tell him or her to be gentle. For an acute case, *do not* massage.

☞ Stand with feet shoulder width apart. Put your hands on your back. Use your palms, or the heel of the palms to scrub up and down from your waist to sacrum 100 times.

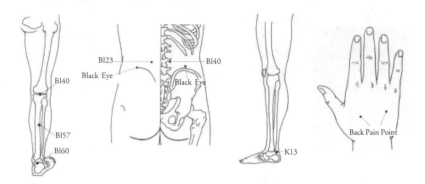

- Stand with feet shoulder width apart. Place your hands on your back just below your waist. Your thumbs are right on two acupressure points, which are called "Back Eyes." Gently press these two points. Meanwhile slowly rotate your body forward, backward, left, and right. Make loose fists and gently tap against this point for one minute.
- Find the most painful spot. Gently tap against the painful spot 30 times. Gently knead for one minute.
- Use your thumb to gently press and knead the point that is a little higher than the waist, two finger-widths on both sides of the spine for one minute (Bl23).
- Lie down on your stomach. Ask a family member to use the thumb to gently press the point in the middle of the crease on the back of the knee for one minute (Bl40).
- Gently press and knead the point in the depression underneath the large muscle, about halfway between the knee crease and the heel for one minute (Bl57).
- Use your thumb and index finger to pinch the dent behind the anklebone on both side, of the foot 10 times (Bl60, Ki3).
- Use your thumb to gently press and knead the point at the back of your hand, two finger-widths from the wrist crease. One is between the ring and middle fingers. Another is between the index and middle fingers ("Back Pain Point"). Do it for one minute.

Chinese Herbs

- Take the patent herb Yu Nan Bai Yao. Follow the instructions.
- Apply the patent herb patch Shang Shi Zhi Tong Gao. If you have an allergic reaction, discontinue use.
- Apply a patent heating patch with herbs, called Chinese Moxibustion. Follow the instructions.

Bed-Wetting

WHAT IS IT AND WHAT CAUSES IT?

Bed-wetting is the involuntary loss of urine during sleep after the age of 5 years, mostly because the urine-filled bladder doesn't wake your child. Genetics, stress, or some underlying diseases may be the causes.

WHEN SHOULD YOU SEE A DOCTOR?

If bed-wetting becomes frequent, or is accompanied with pain or with blood, your child should see a doctor.

WHAT SHOULD YOU DO IN DAILY LIFE?

- Give your child a supportive environment. Blaming won't help. Asking your child to help clean up after bed-wetting may help to some degree.
- Set up a schedule to go to the bathroom, no matter if your child needs to go or not. Then gradually increase the interval time between bathroom visits. Be sure to urinate before bedtime.

WHAT SHOULDN'T YOU DO?

- Don't drink too much at night or before bed.

Folk Remedies

- Pepper on the belly button (navel): Sew a 1-inch square bag with thin cotton fabric. Fill in with some black pepper

powders and seal it. Tape it to the belly button with bandage. Change it every day for one week. If you find any
allergic reaction on the skin, discontinue use.

☞ Take egg with white peppercorn. Open a small hole on
an uncooked egg. Insert seven white peppercorns and
seal it. Steam it until well done. Take two eggs before
bedtime without water for one week. If your child is
younger than 5 years old, only take one egg each time.

Food Therapy

☞ Eating dried litchi can help the bed-wetting. It is an Asian
fruit and available at Chinese grocery stores.

☞ Drink corn silk tea: Place 1 ounce of corn silk in a pot
with 2 cups of water. Bring to a boil and simmer for 10
minutes. Add 1 Tbs. of sugar. Drink once a day for 10
days.

Chinese Massage

☞ Use your thumb and other fingers to *gently* grasp the
muscles right below your child's bellybutton 10 times.
Use your palm to *gently* rub counterclockwise around his
or her belly button until he or she feels warm.

☞ Use your thumb to *gently* press and knead the points a
little higher than the waist, two finger-widths on either
side of the spine for one minute.

☞ You can do the following hand massage for your child:

 ➺ Using the palm surface of your thumb, *gently* push
 along the outside edge of the child's thumb from the
 tip to the root of the thumb. Repeat 100 times.

 ➺ Using the palm surface of your thumb, *gently* push the
 palm surface of the child's ring finger from the tip to
 the transverse (palm root) crease of that ring finger.
 Repeat 100 times.

 ➺ Using the palm surface of your thumb, *gently* push the
 palm surface of the child's little finger from the palm
 root to the tip of that little finger. Repeat 100 times.

⇥ Using your middle finger, *gently* knead the child's hand at the depression between the ring and little fingers on the back of the hand for one minute.

Heat Therapy

Light a smokeless moxa stick, which is like a cigar and available at Chinese herb stores. Circle it one to two inches above the midline between the belly button and pubic bone for 10 minutes. Do this one to two times a day. Be careful not to let the stick or its ashes burn your child.

Breastfeeding Problem 1: Lack of Breast Milk

WHAT IS IT AND WHAT CAUSES IT?

The absence or insufficiency of breast milk during the period of nursing has two causes. If malnutrition and bad physical health are the causes, the breast milk would be very thin. If it is brought on by psychological stress such as anger and depression, breasts would be painful and over-swollen with no milk.

WHEN SHOULD YOU SEE A DOCTOR?

If self-treatments are not working, then you should see a doctor to determine if there are other conditions with mammary ducts.

WHAT SHOULD YOU DO IN DAILY LIFE?

* Before breastfeeding, massage the breast and nipples with a warm and moist towel. This will facilitate the flow of milk.
* When breast milk is plentiful, use a breast pump to extract milk for storage. This will increase the secretion of milk.
* Maintain good nutrition. Drink more soup-type food. Eating more shrimp, pig's feet, sesame seed, pumpkin seed, or dates can help.
* Take enough Vitamin E. It can expand the mammary glands and, therefore, increase the output of milk.

WHAT SHOULDN'T YOU DO?

- Don't give up on breastfeeding because of difficulty. This will only further decrease the amount of breast milk secreted. The act of breastfeeding will stimulate the release.
- Don't exhaust yourself and don't engage in activities that will interfere with your sleep pattern.
- Don't watch horror movies or TV programs that you know will frighten you a lot. Your psychological reactions will have a big impact on your body's processes such as breast milk secretion.
- Don't eat cold and raw food, or ice cream.
- Don't eat food that will decrease the secretion of breast milk such as prickly ash peel or germinated barley.

Folk Remedies

- Apply 6 oz. of self-raising flour dough to the whole breast. Cover with a warm towel for 30 minutes. Take the dough away and use a breast pump to draw the milk out. Massage from the root of the breast to the nipple to help milk flow if necessary.
- Boil 1 oz. of green onions with 2 cups of water. Use the fluids to wash the breast. Wash off with clean water afterwards. Then use a coarse hair comb to gently run it down the breast for 10 minutes, and periodically use the back of the comb to massage the breast. Do so two or three times a day. If your skin is allergic to green onions, don't use this method.

Food Therapy

- Drink fish soup:

    Ingredients: One crucian carp (available in Asian seafood grocery stores), 3 oz. mung bean sprouts, salt.

    Procedure: Add 3 cups of water to ingredients and cook as soup. Eat the fish and drink the soup. Do so once a day for three days.

☞ Drink seaweed with soybean milk:

> **Ingredients:** 1 oz. seaweed, 300 ml soymilk.
>
> **Procedure:** Soak seaweed in water overnight. Wash it clean. Add 2 cups of water to cook seaweed until it is soft. Take it out and mix with soymilk to eat. No salt or sugar. Do so for five days.

☞ Eat pig's feet:

> **Ingredients:** Two fresh pig's feet (available at Chinese grocery stores), 2 oz. soybeans.
>
> **Procedure:** Soak soybeans in water overnight. Place all ingredients in a pot with water to bring to a boil, then simmer for another two hours. Eat the feet and drink the soup every day for three days.

Chinese Massage

Choose the following and massage once a day:

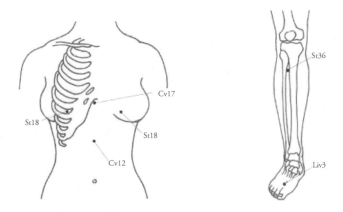

☞ Use your palms to gently rub your left breast clockwise and your right breast couter clockwise for one minute.

☞ Spread your fingers and grasp the breasts. Then gently pull outward and release. Do so for two minutes.

☞ Use your fingertips to gently press against the point right between fourth and fifth ribs on the midline (Cv17) for one minute. Then gently press against the spots directly below each breast (St18) for one minute. Finally, gently press the point halfway between the belly button (navel) and the lower edge of the breastbone for one minute (Cv12).

☞ Gently press the depression four finger-widths below the kneecap edge and a thumb's-width outside of the shin-bone for one mintute (St36).

☞ Gently press the point between the big and second toes, two finger-widths up the foot from the joint between the toes for one minute (Liv3).

Breastfeeding Problems 2: Trouble Stopping the Production of Breast Milk

WHAT IS IT?

You have stopped breastfeeding yet the milk still keeps flowing.

WHAT SHOULD YOU DO IN DAILY LIFE?

☞ Gradually have less frequent breastfeeding to see if the milk will decrease in quantity. If it doesn't, don't stop breastfeeding abruptly.

WHAT SHOULDN'T YOU DO?

☞ Don't eat much animal protein and fat.

Folk Remedies

☞ Boil 2 oz. of germinated barley in water. It is available in Chinese herb stores. Drink as tea once a day for three or four days.

☞ Eat prickly ash peel with sugar:

Ingredients: 1/4 oz. prickly ash peel, brown sugar.

Procedure: Add 1 1/2 cups of water to cook the prickly ash peel until only 3/4 of a cup of water is left. Strain and add sugar to drink. Drink once a day for three days.

☞ Eat dried black beans with rice:

> **Ingredients:** 2 oz. dried black beans (cooking season-ing, available in Chinese grocery stores), 2 oz. rice, 1 Tbs. Chinese cooking oil.
>
> **Procedure:** Cook rice first. Stir-fry rice with black beans and cooking oil for five minutes on low heat. Add a bit of salt to taste. Eat once a day for three days.

Chinese Herbs

☞ Boil 1/8 oz. of senna leaf in one cup of water. Drink as tea twice a day. This may decrease the amount of breast milk. Two days should stop production of breast milk. If you already have loose stool before the treatment, you shouldn't use this method. If you develop loose stool af-ter taking it, stop using it.

Bronchitis

WHAT IS IT AND WHAT CAUSES IT?

It is an inflammation of the airways of the lungs. The symptoms are severe cough with green or yellow phlegm, shortness of breath, and wheezing. Bronchitis is mainly caused by viral or bacterial infection.

In Chinese medicine there are three types of bronchitis:

✻ *Cold Type*: Coughs after you are getting cold, plenty of phlegm, thin and white; running nose, and aversion to cold.

✻ *Heat Type*: Coughs that are frequently and severe, thick and yellow phlegm, shortness of breath or wheezing, and thirst.

✻ *Dry Type*: Dry cough, no phlegm (or very hard to cough up), and dry sore throat and mouth.

WHEN SHOULD YOU SEE A DOCTOR?

If your cough isn't getting better within three days, you have fe-ver, blood in your phlegm, you are elderly, or you have chronic ill-nesses, see a doctor.

WHAT SHOULD YOU DO IN DAILY LIFE?

- Rest if you have fever.
- Drink plenty of water to thin mucus. Particularly, drinking strong green tea will help.
- Eat easily digested foods, such as radish, spinach, tomato, Chinese cabbage, winter melon, soybeans, kelp, orange, pears, dates, water chestnuts, lily bulb, and lotus seed.
- Keep regular aerobic exercise such as walking, jogging, and practicing Tai Chi. Swimming is the best choice for lung-related disease.
- If you have tendency to have bronchitis in winter, adjust yourself to increase the ability to resist cold weather. Wash your face or feet with cold water in summertime.
- Play a woodwind musical instrument to make your chest diaphragm move more actively. This can increase the function of your lungs.
- In chronic cases, you need to have more confidence to fight the disease. A bad psychological factor makes your immune system weak and susceptible to an attack.
- Quit smoking right away. A smoker has much higher risk of getting bronchitis than a non-smoker.
- Keep your room clean and vacuum frequently. Use humidifiers to keep adequate humidity. Keep the air in your room fresh.

WHAT SHOULDN'T YOU DO?

- Don't travel to areas with heavily polluted air.
- Avoid fried food. Avoid seafood such as fish, crab, and shrimp. Don't eat spicy food such as hot pepper, garlic, green onion, mustard, and cinnamon. Don't have milk and dairy products, which may cause more mucus. Don't eat food that is too salty or too sweet.
- If you have upper respiratory problems, don't delay treatments.

Folk Remedies

☞ Use a hairbrush to tap the lung meridians for three minutes before bedtime. They are found on the inner side, from top of both arms down to the tips of your thumbs. Tap only along this direction. Do it for a prolonged period. The brush's needles stimulate all the points on your lung meridian and make it like an acupuncture treatment.

☞ Inhale warm air from vinegar: Pour 1 cup of white rice vinegar into a pot and bring to a simmer on low heat. Pour the vinegar into a thermos. Use a funnel as a lid to cover the thermos. Sitting in front of the thermos, inhale the warm air from vinegar for 20 minutes. Continue to do it for a week. Take care not to burn yourself.

Food Therapy

☞ Drink green tea with egg:

Ingredients: 2 eggs, 1/2 oz. green tea leaves, 3 oz. brown sugar.

Procedure: Place green tea leaves into a pot. Add 2 cups of water, and bring to a boil. Add eggs and sugar and cook until the eggs are medium done. Use a spoon to break the eggshells. Let the tea totally penetrate into the egg. Continue to decoct until only one cup of liquid is remaining. Remove shells. Eat eggs and drink the soup once a day. Repeat this procedure everyday for a week.

☞ Eat egg with honey:

Ingredients: 1 egg, honey.

Procedure: Crack the egg into a bowl. Add 1/2 cup of water and 1 Tbs. of honey. Beat and mix well. Steam for five minutes. Eat twice a day, more frequently in wintertime.

☞ Eat radish with lotus and pear:

Ingredients: 1/2 lb. radish, 1/2 lb. lotus root, 2 Asian pears, ginger, honey.

Procedure: Place radish, lotus root, and pears into a juicer to make juice. Add 1 Tbs. of honey. Steam for five minutes. Add 2 to 3 drops of ginger juice. Divide into two portions. Drink twice a day for a week.

☞ If you have the cold-type bronchitis, take sweet apricot seed with sugar:

Ingredients: 1/8 oz. sweet apricot seeds (available in Chinese herb stores), 1 tsp. brown sugar.

Procedure: Smash into small pieces. Soak them in 1 cup of hot water with 1 tsp. honey. Drink it as tea.

☞ If you have the heat-type bronchitis, drink olive tea with radish:

Ingredients: 3 oz. olive, 3 oz. daikon radish.

Procedure: Add 3 cups of water and ingredients to a pot and bring to a boil. Reduce heat and simmer for 10 minutes. Drink it as tea.

☞ If you have the dry-type bronchitis, drink the following tea:

Ingredients: 1 oz. fresh lily bulb, 1/2 oz. sweet apricot seeds, 2 oz. rice, 1 Tbs. sugar.

Procedure: Cut the tip of the apricot seeds out. Add 3 cups of water and rice to a pot, bring to a boil. Reduce heat and simmer for 15 minutes. Then add lily bulb, apricot seed, and sugar. Cook for another five minutes. Divide into two portions. Drink twice a day.

Chinese Massage

Choose from the following and massage once a day:

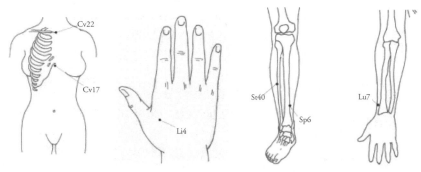

☞ Use the tips of the index, middle, and ring fingers of both hands to scrub up and down the center of the breastbone for one minute. Gently press and knead the breastbone from the top to the bottom for one minute.

☞ Gently press and knead the point right in the middle between the nipples for men, and between fourth and fifth ribs on the midline for women (Cv17). Do this for one minute.

☞ Gently press the point located at the depression right above the top of the breastbone for one minute (Cv22). Use your fingers to gently squeeze the skin and muscles from this point up to the Adam's apple 20 times.

☞ With your thumb against the index finger, use your other thumb to gently press the webbing where it bulges up the highest for one minute (Li4).

☞ Gently press the point located two finger-widths up from the wrist crease, on the inside of the forearm, in line with the thumb, for one minute (Lu7).

☞ Gently press the point on the outside edge of the leg bone halfway between the tip of the anklebone and the middle of the kneecap for one minute (St40).

☞ Gently press the point four finger-widths up from the inside anklebone, right behind the leg bone for one minute (Sp6).

Chinese Herbs

☞ If you have cold-type bronchitis, take the patent herb Tong Xuan Li Fei Wan. Follow the instructions.

☞ If you have heat-type bronchitis, drink the patent herb She Dan Chuan Bei Ye. Follow the instructions.

☞ If you have dry-type cough bronchitis, take the patent herb Yang Yin Qing Fei Wan. Follow the instructions.

☞ Eat Asian pear with herb:

> **Ingredients:** 1 Asian pear, 1/8 oz. tendrilled fritillary bulb.
>
> **Procedure:** Cut a small opening on the pear. Remove the seeds. Place the herb inside. Steam for 40 minutes. Eat the pear once a day.

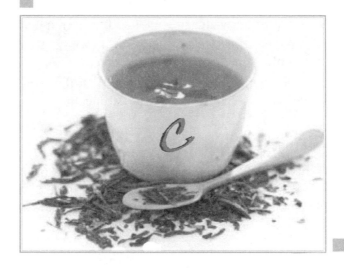

Calluses and Corns

WHAT IS IT AND WHAT CAUSES IT?

Calluses and corns are thick layers of dead skin that are the result of excessive pressure and friction. They can occur anywhere, but most commonly appear on your hands and feet.

WHEN SHOULD YOU SEE A DOCTOR?

If your calluses or corns affect you daily, see a doctor. If you have diabetes and also suffer from calluses or corns on your feet, see a doctor.

WHAT SHOULD YOU DO IN DAILY LIFE?

* Wear comfortable and well-fitting shoes. It's best to have up to three pairs of comfortable shoes to exchange and not wear one pair all the time.

WHAT SHOULDN'T YOU DO?

* Don't try to cut away the corn by yourself.

Folk Remedies

- ☞ Scrape the corns with a small and smooth pebble once a day.
- ☞ Use warm to hot water to soak feet for 30 minutes a day, (10 minutes, three times a day) for a month. Be careful not to burn yourself.
- ☞ Carve out a small indentation larger than the corn inside of your shoes where the calluses rub against it.

Chinese Massage

- ☞ Wash your feet with warm water. When you are watching TV, gently caresse the callused area as long as possible. Do so for a prolonged period.

Chinese Herbs

- ☞ Apply herb paste:

    Ingredients: Wolfberry bark, safflower, sesame oil.

    Procedure: Grind to a fine powder. Mix with sesame oil and apply to affected area for five hours a day.

Canker Sores

WHAT IS IT AND WHAT CAUSES IT?

It is an ulcer surrounded by red swelling in the mouth. The precise cause of canker sores is still not determined, though multiple reasons, such as stress, physical trauma, and bacterial infection, may contribute to it.

WHEN SHOULD YOU SEE A DOCTOR?

If the canker sores do not improve for a long period of time or if you have recurrent sores, see a doctor.

WHAT SHOULD YOU DO IN DAILY LIFE?

- ☞ Maintain good oral hygiene.
- ☞ Eat more vegetables and fruits.

- Have regular bowel movements.
- Control your emotions.

WHAT SHOULDN'T YOU DO?

- Don't consume overstimulating items such as spicy or fried food. Don't eat fish.
- Don't drink alcohol and caffeine.

Folk Remedies

- Crush Vitamin C pills and apply it on sores. Do so twice a day for three days. At the same time, take 200 mg of Vitamin C three times a day. If you have an allergic reaction, discontinue use.
- Cut out an aloe vera leaf and apply the liquid on the sores. Do so three times a day for two or three days. If you have an allergic reaction stop.
- Slowly chew 1 tsp. soaked green tea leaves.

Food Therapy

- Soak 2 oz. of mung beans and 1 oz. of lotus seeds in water overnight. Place them in a pot with 3 cups of water and cook until they are soft. Add one beaten egg to the pot. Cook for another 20 seconds. Take twice a day.
- Frequently hold watermelon juice in your mouth for three minutes, then swallow. Or use radish juice to rinse your mouth three times a day.

Chinese Herbs

- Apply the patent herb powder Shuang Liao Hou Feng San. Follow the instructions.
- If canker sores keep recurring, try the patent herb pill Zhi Bai Di Huang Wan. Follow the instructions.

Carpal Tunnel Syndrome

WHAT IS IT AND WHAT CAUSES IT?

It is the numbness or tingling and pain in the fingers. The pain may radiate to the palms, wrists, and forearms. Carpal tunnel is a gap where some nerves and tendons pass through to arrive at the hand. When tendons have an inflammation, the space becomes too crowded. The hand numbness and pain occur if the nerve is pressed.

WHEN SHOULD YOU SEE A DOCTOR?

If the pain affects your daily life, see a doctor.

WHAT SHOULD YOU DO IN DAILY LIFE?

- When your hand starts tingling, rotate your wrist for a minute.
- If your wrist is swelling, apply an ice pack or a bag of frozen beans wrapped with a cloth to your arm for 15 to 20 minutes three to four times a day.
- When you lie down, elevate your arm with pillows to relieve the discomfort.
- If you work with a computer frequently, your fingers should be lower than your wrist. Keep your wrist straight. Don't flex. Type with a soft touch. Take breaks during long periods of work. Keep your palms facing up or sit with your elbows supported on the desk when you take a rest.
- Wear a splint when you are working with your hands for prolonged periods.

WHAT SHOULDN'T YOU DO?

- Don't grip the wheel too tightly when driving.
- Don't eat much salt, which causes water retention and promotes swelling.
- Don't smoke, which constricts the small blood vessels.

Folk Remedies

☞ In a chronic case, wrap leaves of cabbage around your wrist: Cut the hard rib out of a dark green cabbage leaf. Warm it in microwave until it becomes soft. Wrap it around your wrist and fix with a bandage.

☞ In a chronic case, blow the pain away: Set a low-power hair dryer at low. Blow the warm air on the forearm and hand from the distance you can feel warm air for two minutes, twice a day. This treatment is only for chronic cases. Take care not to burn yourself.

☞ In a chronic case, wash with vinegar:

> **Ingredients:** 500 ml rice vinegar, 6 inches of green onion.
>
> **Procedure:** Warm up vinegar and onion. Wash the forearm, wrist, and hand with this liquid for 10 minutes. Reheat if necessary. Discontinue use if you have an allergic reaction.

Food Therapy

☞ Drink warm red wine: Use a microwave to warm 30 ml red wine. Drink twice a day.

Chinese Massage

In chronic cases, choose the following and massage once a day:

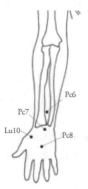
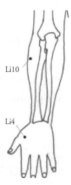

- Using the heel of your palm to rub and knead both sides of the wrist and the two big bones in your forearm for one minute. Meanwhile gently bend and flex the wrist.
- Using the thumb and four fingers grasp the muscles from your forearm to your fingers for one minute. With your thumb against the index finger, use your other thumb and index finger to grasp the webbing where it bulges up the highest for one minute (Li4).
- Using your thumb, gently press and knead each of the following points for one minute:
  - The point two thumb-widths above the wrist crease of the palm side, between the tendons, right under the buckle of the watchstrap (Pc6).
  - On the center of your palm, where the middle finger touches when you are making a fist (Pc8).
  - The middle of the crease between the tendons on the palm side (Pc7).
  - The point on the pad of the thumb two finger-widths from the wrist, on the borderline between the dark and light skin (Lu10).
  - On the forearm two thumb-widths below the crease of the elbow in line with the thumb (Li10).

Chinese Herbs

- Rub the patent tincture Zheng Gu Shui to painful spots. Follow the instructions. If you have an allergic reaction, discontinue use.
- Take the patent herb Yu Nan Bai Yao. Follow the instructions.
- Apply the herb patch Shang Shi Zhi Tong Gao. Follow the instructions. If you have an allergic reaction, discontinue use.

Cataracts

WHAT IS IT AND WHAT CAUSES IT?

Cataracts cause vision blurring or dimming because the lenses of your eyes become cloudy and opaque. Other symptoms are double vision, halos or sensitiveness around lights, and poor color perception. In severe cases your lens may look milky white or yellowish. Along with aging, diabetes, overexposure to ultraviolet light, smoking, and heredity can be the causes.

WHEN SHOULD YOU SEE A DOCTOR?

If you have any vision problems, see an eye specialist.

WHAT SHOULD YOU DO IN DAILY LIFE?

- ⋇ Wear ultraviolet-protective sunglasses if necessary.
- ⋇ Research shows people who drink at least 5 cups of green tea a day can reduce the risk of cataracts.
- ⋇ Take enough vitamins C and vitamin E.
- ⋇ Eat more zinc-rich food such as peanuts, sesame seeds, bean products, fish, and shrimp.

WHAT SHOULDN'T YOU DO?

- ⋇ Don't expose yourself to strong light, high temperatures, or chemical solutions for prolonged periods of time.
- ⋇ Do not read books or watch TV for longer than one hour.
- ⋇ Don't use halogen lights, as they cause the pupils to constrict.
- ⋇ Don't eat fried food or too many sweets.
- ⋇ Don't smoke.

Folk Remedies

- ☞ Walk with bare feet at home as much as you can. Place five golf balls in a plastic shallow container. Sit on a chair and roll these balls with your soles for 20 minutes a day.
- ☞ Dip a washcloth in water as hot as is comfortable for your skin. Wring out the excess water and cover your eyes and forehead. Change to a new one when it becomes cool. Repeat 10 times until your head feels warm. Do this every morning.

Food Therapy

☞ Drink white chrysanthemum tea:

Ingredients: 1/4 oz. white chrysanthemum.

Procedure: Add chrysanthemum to 1 1/2 cups of water and bring to a boil. Reduce heat and simmer for 10 minutes. Strain the decoction to drink, once a day.

☞ Drink green peas and corn soup:

Ingredients: 2 oz. green peas, 2 oz. corn.

Procedure: Add the green peas and corn to 2 cups of water and salt to make soup. Drink once a day.

☞ Drink soybean milk with black sesame and walnuts:

Ingredients: 1/2 oz. black sesame seeds, 1/2 oz. walnuts, 300 ml soybean milk, honey.

Procedure: Stir-fry sesame seeds and walnuts on low heat for two minutes. Grind them, then add to soybean milk. Add 1 tsp. of honey. Take once every day.

☞ Eat black beans, black dates, dried white beans:

Ingredients: 1 oz. black beans, 10 black dates, 1 oz. dried white beans, available at Chinese grocery stores.

Procedure: Soak beans in water overnight. Add enough water to cover all ingredients. Bring to a boil. Reduce heat and simmer until beans are soft. Eat as a snack every afternoon.

Chinese Massage

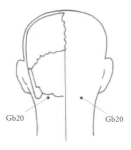
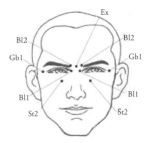

- ☞ Eye exercise:
    - ⮞ Rub your palms against each other until they are warm. Place the center of your palms right over your eyeballs to feel a warm sensation in your eyes. Repeat this 10 times.
    - ⮞ Close your eyes for five seconds. Quickly open. Repeat several times.
    - ⮞ Close your eyes. Move your eyeballs in a clockwise circle five times. Move them in a counterclockwise circle five times.
    - ⮞ Use the pad of both thumbs to gently press and knead the following area: from the frame of eyes, the temple, above the ears, to the back of your head. Do this for two minutes.
- ☞ Gently press and knead each point for one minute once a day:
    - ⮞ The points in the depression, half a thumb's-width outside the corner of the eye (Gb1).
    - ⮞ The point one finger-width right below the eye socket in line with the pupil (St2).
    - ⮞ The depression right at the inner corner of your eyes (Bl1).
    - ⮞ The middle point of your eyebrows (EX).
    - ⮞ The point in the depression on the beginning of the eyebrow (Bl2).
    - ⮞ The point in the depression at the bottom of the skull, outside of the two big muscles on the neck, which you can feel by bending down your neck (Gb20).

Chinese Herbs

- ☞ Eat lycium with longan aril:

    Ingredients: 1/4 oz. lycium fruit, 5 longan arils (Asian fruit). Both are available in Chinese grocery stores.

    Procedure: Add fruits and 1 cup of water to a pot and bring to a boil. Reduce heat and simmer for 10 minutes. Eat once a day.

Cholesterol (High)

WHAT IS IT AND WHAT CAUSES IT?

High cholesterol means that the fat in your bloodstream has problems. You have too much LDL (low density lipoprotein), the "bad' cholesterol. It can deposit on blood vessels and add to risk for heart disease, stroke, and vascular disorders. Also, you may lack HDL (high density lipoprotein), the good cholesterol. It clears cholesterol out from your body. High cholesterol level is mainly caused by rich diet or genetic problems.

WHEN SHOULD YOU SEE A DOCTOR?

You should get tested on a regular basis. If a child has a family history of high cholesterol or cardiovascular disease, he or she needs to see a doctor.

WHAT SHOULD YOU DO IN DAILY LIFE?

- Change your eating habits. If you don't eat breakfast and eat too much for dinner, your cholesterol will be much higher than those who eat three regular meals a day. Be sure to eat a good breakfast. Eat lightly. Stop eating when you feel 70-percent full and you will live much longer.

- Watch what you eat very carefully.
  - Be aware that eggs, animal organs, cheese, pork fat, and western-style desserts have much high cholesterol.
  - Eat omega-3 rich food and soluble fiber. Mostly eat fish and vegetables such as mushrooms, celery, carrots, corn, sweet potato, peanuts, walnuts, and whole grains. Also eat garlic, onion, soybeans, hawthorn berries, mung beans, tofu, Chinese dry mushrooms, sunflower seeds, red dates, and kelp. Eat fruits such as kiwi, apples, and oranges.
  - Drink green tea such as Wu Long tea.
  - Drink wine moderately.
  - Add rice vinegar to your diet.

> ✹ Exercise regularly. Research shows exercise can raise good cholesterol level and lower bad cholesterol level.

WHAT SHOULDN'T YOU DO?

> ✹ Never eat or drink too much at a time.
> ✹ Don't smoke.
> ✹ Don't live a stressful life, which could make your cholesterol higher.

Folk Remedies

> ☞ Take 1/8 oz. red rice yeast powder a day.

Food Therapy

> ☞ Eat garlic 1/4 oz. at a time, twice a day. If you feel it makes your stomach uncomfortable stop. Or eat one kiwi a day. Or eat sunflower seeds, 1/2 oz., once a day. Continue for one month.
> ☞ Eat peanuts with vinegar:
>   **Ingredients:** Rice vinegar, peanuts with red skin.
>   **Procedure:** Soak peanuts in vinegar for 10 days. Eat 10 to 15 pieces at a time, twice a day.
>
> ☞ Eat red bell pepper juice:
>   **Ingredients:** 2 red bell peppers.
>   **Procedure:** Cut the peppers in half. Remove the seeds. Use a juicer with 1/2 cup of water to make pepper juice. Add a few drops of olive oil. Eat 2 Tbs. at a time, twice a day for a prolonged period.
>
> ☞ Eat black and white fungus with crystal sugar:
>   **Ingredients:** 1/4 oz. black fungus, 1/4 oz. white fungus, 1/4 oz. crystal sugar. These items are available from Chinese grocery stores.
>   **Procedure:** Soak fungus in warm water for three hours. Wash and clean them carefully. Place in a bowl. Add one cup of water and sugar. Steam for one hour. Eat the fungus and drink the soup.

☞ Eat kelp with mung bean:

Ingredients: 1/2 oz. kelp (dried seaweed), 1/2 oz. mung beans, 1/2 oz. brown sugar.

Procedure: Soak kelp and mung beans in water overnight. Slice kelp into inch-long pieces. Add 3 cups of water and kelp to a pot and bring to a boil. Reduce heat and simmer until the beans are soft. Divide into two portions. Eat with sugar, twice a day.

Chinese Herbs

☞ Take 1/16 oz. of pseudoginseng powder at a time, two times a day.

☞ Drink lycium fruit tea: Steep 1/4 oz. of lycium fruit in boiled water. Drink as tea.

Cold (Common) and Flu

WHAT IS IT AND WHAT CAUSES IT?

The common cold is an upper respiratory infection caused by a cold virus. The symptoms include runny nose, sneezing, sore throat, coughing, and possibly fever. Flu has almost all the above symptoms and is caused by a flu virus. It is hard to distinguish between flu and cold, except that the person suffering from flu may have a higher fever.

There are three types of colds in Chinese medicine:

✦ *Cold Type*: Aversion to cold, no sweating, sneezing, low-grade fever, white and thin mucus, and cough. It often occurs in winter or spring.

✦ *Heat Type*: Fever, sweating, sore or itching throat, dry mouth and nose, cough, yellowish and thick mucus or nose discharge. It often occurs in later spring or the beginning of fall.

✦ *Damp Type*: Fever, head heaviness, nausea, and bloating in chest or lower abdomen. It often happens in the hot summer season.

WHEN SHOULD YOU SEE A DOCTOR?

If you have a high fever or your fever lasts for more than two or three days, or if you feel a severe pain in the ear, stomach, lungs, or head, see your doctor. If you have swollen tonsils or neck glands and have developed rapid breathing or wheezing, see a doctor.

WHAT SHOULD YOU DO IN DAILY LIFE?

- Drink plenty of water or green tea. Drink 8 cups of water a day.
- Eat easily digested food. Eat more garlic and onion , and zinc-rich foods, such as milk, soymilk, lean meats, fish, beans, and cheese.
- If you can take care of the following you are much less likely to get colds:
  - Keep your body warm, especially your feet. Watch for change of weather. If you get wet in rain, drink hot tea with five ginger slices and 1 tsp. of brown sugar.
  - Take it easy. Don't be exhausted by anything.
  - Get enough sleep.
  - Washing your hands frequently can prevent a cold.
  - During summertime wash your face and nose with cold water. Gradually advance to taking a cold shower if possible.
- In flu season, use salt water to rinse your mouth (1 tsp. of salt with 8 oz. of water), or hold a salty olive in your mouth when you have to go outside.
- Keep your room moist and warm with fresh air. During flu season, fumigate your room with vinegar. Add 50 ml rice vinegar to 50 ml water for each 100 feet^2. Heat on stove to sterilize the air.

WHAT SHOULDN'T YOU DO?

- Avoid spicy, salty, and greasy food. Avoid raw, cold food. Don't eat watermelon or cucumber if you feel you are going to catch cold. Don't drink alcohol.
- Don't go to sleep right after washing your hair. Wait until the hair is dry.

- Avoid public places as much as possible.
- Avoid vigorously blowing your nose to prevent an ear infection. Blow one nostril at a time. If you have a cold, don't go on an airplane.

Folk Remedies

- Boil 250 ml rice vinegar, and soak a washcloth inside. Place the washcloth under your nose and inhale the warm vinegar for two minutes. Be careful to not burn yourself.
- Cover your mouth and nose with a warm wet washcloth. Set a hair dryer to low and blow hot air on your face for one minute. Keep the washcloth wet and warm. Do this three times a day. Take care not to scald yourself.
- Use a pair of tongs to hold a tangerine. Heat on top of the stove. Turn over continuously until you smell strong fragrance. Peel, but keep the tangerine pith. Eat it at the beginning of your cold.
- Applying toothpaste on both temples and the groove below the nose, slightly more then halfway up, may relieve symptoms.

Food Therapy

- Drink garlic milk:

   Ingredients: 1 clove garlic, milk.

   Procedure: Peel garlic, pound to small pieces. Add 1 cup of hot milk to a pot. Stir and soak for 15 minutes. Use a piece of gauze to filter the garlic out of the milk when pouring it out of the pot. Slowly drink the milk, three times a day. Stop if garlic makes your stomach upset.

- Eat radish with green onion:

   Ingredients: 6 oz. radish, 3 white stalks of green onion.

   Procedure: Add ingredients to 3 cups of water and bring to a boil. Reduce heat and simmer for 10 minutes. Eat radish and drink soup once a day.

❧ Drink green tea with mung bean:

> **Ingredients:** 1 oz. mung beans, 1/4 oz. green tea, 1 oz. sugar.
>
> **Procedure:** Soak mung beans in water overnight. Place green tea in a gauze bag. Place both tea and beans in a pot and add 3 cups of water. Bring to a boil. Reduce heat and simmer until beans are soft. Add sugar. Eat beans and drink soup once a day.

Chinese Massage

Choose from the following and massage once a day:

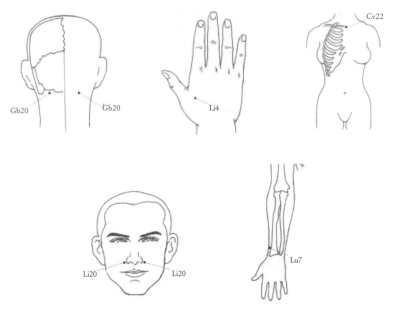

❧ Rub your hands against each other until they are warm. Use both palms to gently rub your face from the forehead down to the chin, from the temples down to the lower jaw until your face feels warm.

❧ Use the index and middle fingers to push from the central point between your eyebrows to both temples for one minute.

- ☞ Use your four fingers to repeatedly rub the back of the head. Also repeatedly rub the point in the depression at the bottom of the skull, outside of the two big muscles on the neck, which you can feel by bending down your neck (Gb20).
- ☞ With your thumb against the index finger, use your other thumb to gently press the webbing where it bulges up the highest for one minute (Li4).
- ☞ Gently press the point located two finger-widths up from the wrist crease, on the inside of the forearm, in line with the thumb for one minute (Lu7).
- ☞ If your nose is congested, use the index finger to gently press the point in the middle of the groove of the outside edge of the nostril for one minute (Li20). Using your thumb and index finger rub and knead from the inner corner of your eyes down to the bottom of your nose for one minute.
- ☞ If you are coughing, gently press the depression right above the top of the breastbone for one minute (Cv22).

Chinese Herbs

- ☞ If you have heat-type, take the patent herb Yin Qiao Jie Du Pian. Follow the instructions.
- ☞ If you have cold-type, take the patent herb Gan Mao Qing Re Chong Ji. Follow the instructions.
- ☞ If you have damp-type, take the patent herb Huo Xiang Zheng Qi Shui. Follow the instructions.

Colic

WHAT IS IT AND WHAT CAUSES IT?

It is the persistent crying of a baby with no apparent health problems. The cause of periodic and intense outbursts can be hard to decipher because babies have no other way to communicate their discomfort.

WHEN SHOULD YOU SEE A DOCTOR?

The persistent crying may be a sign of an underlying health problem. You should take your baby to the doctor at any signs of colic.

WHAT SHOULD YOU DO IN DAILY LIFE?

- ☙ Feed your baby in an upright position, and burp often. If bottle-feeding, burp the baby after every ounce.
- ☙ Carefully observe your baby. He or she may be hungry, too warm, have insect bites, have a stuffy nose, and so on.

WHAT SHOULDN'T YOU DO?

- ☙ As a breastfeeding mother, you shouldn't eat anything spicy or anything containing caffeine. Eat few bananas, tomatoes, oranges and strawberries. Such food may have an indirect impact on your baby if you are breastfeeding. Stop eating them for five days to see if the crying gets better. Do the same test for dairy products too.
- ☙ Don't feed your baby too much before bedtime.

Folk Remedies

- ☙ Record the baby's cries. When he or she cries again, play the tape back to him or her.
- ☙ Boil an egg and leave the shell intact. Let the egg cool until it is only warm. Touch the egg on your skin to test whether the temperature is comfortable for your baby. If it is, place the egg on the bellybutton and roll it outward in a spiral pattern and then roll it inward.
- ☙ Apply warm salt: Stir-fry 3 oz. of salt until warm. Add 2 oz. of white stalks of green onions. Continue to stir-fry for one minute. Put in a 3 x 3-inch cotton fabric bag (remember to test temperature on your skin) and apply to your baby's abdomen for five minutes before bedtime. Take great care not to burn him or her.
- ☙ Wrap the baby in a blanket.

Chinese Massage

Do the following massage a half hour before bedtime. Use some massage oil on your baby's skin.

- ☞ Use the tip of your nail to *gently* press the central point at the heel of the baby's palm five times. Use your middle finger to *gently* knead the same point 100 times. Do so for both hands.

- ☞ Use both hands to *gently* rub-roll the first joint of your baby's fingers 30 times. Repeat both hands.

- ☞ If your baby has cold limbs, cold lower abdomen, and a greenish stool, use your thumb to *gently* push his or her forearm on the inner side in a line with the thumb from the wrist to the elbow 100 times. Do both arms.

- ☞ If your baby is irritable and has a reddish face, hot hands and a hot abdomen, use your index finger to *gently* push his or her forearm on the inside along the midline from the wrist to the elbow 100 times. Do both arms.

- ☞ If your baby is startled and irritable during sleep, suddenly crying and screaming, use your thumb's nail to *gently* pinch the point at the central point of the second crease of his or her wrist on the palm side five times. Knead that point 100 times. Do both hands.

- ☞ If your baby has poor appetite, reflux, bloated abdomen, *gently* rub his or her lower abdomen for five minutes. Before you massage the abdomen, rub your hands against each other until they are warm. Do this three times a day.

Constipation

WHAT IS IT AND WHAT CAUSES IT?

Constipation is infrequent bowel movements with a dry, hard stool. The main cause is insufficient fiber in your diet. Lack of exercise and fluids in the body are other possible causes.

WHEN SHOULD YOU SEE A DOCTOR?

If you experience constipation for more than five days, or you have a fever, abdominal cramping, or bloody stool, see a doctor.

WHAT SHOULD YOU DO IN DAILY LIFE?

- ⋈ Set a regular bathroom time. Even if you can't have a bowel movement. The best time is 20 minutes after break-fast. Before you go to the bathroom, drink 2 cups of water and walk for 10 minutes.
- ⋈ Eat more fruits and vegetables. Eat more fiber-rich food such as soybeans, yams, sweat potatoes, or celery. Eat more walnuts, honey, sesame seeds, or peanuts to lubricate your intestines. Eat more beans, potatoes, onion, or radish to produce more gas to accelerate the movement of the intestines.
- ⋈ Drink at least 8 cups of water a day.
- ⋈ Take warm baths to increase blood circulation and for personal hygiene in the anus area.
- ⋈ Keep regular exercise. Lack of exercise is the main reason for constipation in the elderly.
- ⋈ If you have hemorrhoids or anal fissures, treat them promptly.

WHAT SHOULDN'T YOU DO?

- ⋈ If you are elderly, don't force your bowel movements.
- ⋈ Don't eat too many dairy products or too much meat or eggs.
- ⋈ Don't ignore the urge to defecate.

Folk Remedies

- ☞ Soak a towel in hot water and place it under your anus for one or two minutes to stimulate the bowels.
- ☞ Watch comedy shows frequently. Laughing functions to massage your intestines.
- ☞ When sitting on the toilet, do the following to accelerate the movement of the intestines:

- Alternately expand and contract your belly through breathing in and out.
- Find the point on the back of the forearm, four finger-widths up from the crease on the wrist (Te6). Use the nail to gently press that point between two bones for one minute.
- Use your left index finger to gently press the point two thumb-widths to the left of the belly button (St25) until you have a sensation of soreness and distention, and continue to press 20 to 30 seconds.

Food Therapy

- Eat fruit or vegetables:
  - Eat one ripe banana and a cup of cold water with 1 tsp. of honey in the morning.
  - Eat 1/2 lb. of yams two to three times a week.
  - Eat a raw cucumber with 1 cup of water on an empty stomach every morning.
- Eat more nuts:
  - Eat 1 oz. of walnuts before bedtime daily for a chronic case.
  - Eat pine seeds. Stir-fry pine seeds lightly. Peel them. Eat 1/2 oz. at a time, twice a day. It is good for the elderly.
- Drink potato juice:

  Ingredients: One baseball-size potato, 1 tsp. honey.

  Procedure: Use a juicer to make potato juice. Mix potato juice and honey with 1/2 cup of cold water and take in the morning on an empty stomach.

Chinese Massage

In daily life, do the following massage to improve the function of your digestive system.

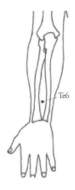 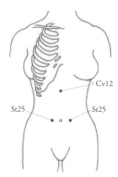

- Lie down and bend your knees up (feet flat on the floor) to relax the muscles on the abdomen. Rub your hands against each other until they are warm. Rub your upper abdomen clockwise 30 times. Rub the lower abdomen clockwise 30 times. Place the right palm on your right lower abdomen and push up. Then push horizontally to left and pass through your belly button. Then push downwards to the pubic bone. Repeat this 10 times.

- Use the pad of your thumb to scrub the area around your waist two finger-widths on both sides of the spine for one minute.

- Use your middle finger to gently press and knead 30 times on the point halfway between the belly button and the lower edge of the breastbone (Cv12).

- Use the middle finger of left hand to gently press and knead 30 times on the point two thumb-widths from your belly button on either side (St25).

Qi Gong

- In the morning before breakfast, stand naturally, with two arms lifted backward, your two palms facing towards the back. Place feet shoulder width apart. Fold your fists forcefully. Meanwhile, inhale and tighten your anus (constrict and lift the anus). Keep this position for two seconds. Then exhale and relax your anus muscles and fists. Repeat this process 30 times. You can also do this exercise on your bed for five minutes every morning.

Chinese Herbs

☞ Take the patent herb honey ball Ma Ren Run Chang Wan. Follow the instructions.

Cough

WHAT IS IT AND WHAT CAUSES IT?

Coughing is a reflex symptom resulting from irritation or excess mucus of the respiratory tract. Cold and flu are the most common causes. There are three types of coughs in Chinese medicine:

- *Cold Type*: Loud cough, thin white phlegm, aversion to cold, and no sweating. It happens in winter or early spring.
- *Heat Type*: Frequent cough with heavy breath, hoarseness, and thick, yellow phlegm. It happens in late spring or early summer.
- *Dry Type*: Dry cough with itching and dry throat, no mucus or it is hard to come out. It happens in late summer or early fall.

WHEN SHOULD YOU SEE A DOCTOR?

If you have a cough for more than three days, or you have a fever, or yellow, green, or bloody mucus, see a doctor.

WHAT SHOULD YOU DO IN DAILY LIFE?

- Drink plenty of water. Drinking hot green tea is a very good choice.
- Keep your body warm. Pay close attention to weather changes.

WHAT SHOULDN'T YOU DO?

⋈ Don't eat raw, cold food. Avoid fat and spicy food. Avoid food that is too sweet or too salty. Avoid seafood.

⋈ Don't overuse cough suppressants.

⋈ Quit smoking right away. Drink less alcohol.

Food Therapy

☞ If you have heat-type cough, drink pear and lotus soup:

Ingredients: 1 Asian pear, 8 oz. lotus root, 1 oz. sugar.

Procedure: Peel the skin off the pear and remove the center. Cut the node of lotus out. Place them in a juicer to make juice. Add sugar and drink once a day.

☞ If you have cold-type cough, drink radish soup:

Ingredients: 6 oz. daikon radish, 3 white stalks of green onion, 1/2 oz. ginger.

Procedure: Add ingredients and 3 cups of water to a pot and cook for five minutes. Drink once a day.

☞ If you have dry-type cough eat walnut and pine nut seeds with honey:

Ingredients: 1 oz. pine nut seeds, 1 oz. walnuts, 15 ml white honey.

Procedure: Pound nuts into small pieces. Mix with honey. Eat 1/4 oz. with warm water after a meal once a day.

☞ If you have a cough for a prolonged period, eat tofu with sugar and ginger:

Ingredients: 8 oz. tofu, 2 oz. sugar, 1/4 oz. ginger.

Procedure: Add ingredients and 2 cups of water to a pot and cook for five minutes. Eat all before bedtime for a week.

☞ If you have a cough for a prolonged period, eat eggs with vinegar:

> **Ingredients:** 70 ml rice vinegar, 3 eggs, 30 ml sesame oil.
> **Procedure:** Beat eggs and scramble in oil. Add vinegar and cook for three minutes. Divide into two portions. Eat twice a day.

Chinese Massage

See **Bronchitis** section.

Chinese Herbs

☞ If you have a cold-type cough, take the patent herb Tong Xuang Li Fei Wan. Follow the instructions.

☞ If you have a heat-type cough, drink the patent herb tincture She Dan Chuan Bei Ye. Follow the instructions.

☞ If you have a dry-type cough, take the patent herb Pi Ba Ye Gao. Follow the instructions.

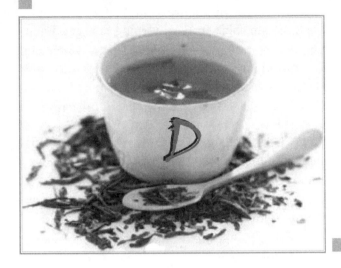

Depression

WHAT IS IT AND WHAT CAUSES IT?

This condition is characterized by a general feeling of sadness and despair. Other signs are insomnia and withdrawal from usual activities. Diseases, psychological trauma, and prolonged stress can all cause depression. Here we focus on depression caused by stress.

WHEN SHOULD YOU CALL A DOCTOR?

Similar to mood disorders such as anxiety, the threshold to seek medical help can be ambiguous. When depression affects your life, see a doctor.

WHAT SHOULD YOU DO IN DAILY LIFE?

* Get sufficient sleep. Soak your feet in warm water for 10 minutes before bedtime to help you go to sleep.
* Regular exercise plays a very important role for depression treatment. It makes your body produce certain chemicals to lift your mood. Also, exercise makes you

have a feeling that you have accomplished a mission and you are still in control. This will compromise the frustrating feeling of the depression. A fast 30-minute walk toward the sunshine in the morning is a good choice.

❦ Try to overcome the feeling of jealousy, which can cause a lot emotional problems and form a vicious cycle. It is an emotion worse than anger.

❦ Eat nutritious food particularly calcium-rich and amino acid-rich food such as milk, bean products, fish, shrimp, chicken, beef, bananas, or dates. The lack of certain vitamins or minerals can contribute to a depressive mood.

❦ Reach out. Join some kind of social activities.

❦ Stand in front of a mirror and smile to yourself for at least one minute twice a day.

❦ Be aware that some medications cause depression. Consult with your doctor.

WHAT SHOULDN'T YOU DO?

❦ Do not suppress your feelings. Find someone you trust very much and pour out your heart to him or her. Let out your emotions and cry if the urge arises. Emotional release is a good, natural necessity in mental health. When you share with others, the toxicity disappears.

❦ Don't talk about any sad topic during your meals. Don't do any intellectual work 20 minutes before or after the meal.

Folk Remedies

❦ With a short sentence, write down on a piece of paper all the frustrations, annoyances, and hatreds that plague you. Repeat the short sentence as many times as you can. After you've finished, burn the paper and watch it crumble into dust (be cautious and perhaps do the burning outdoors). Bring the dust to a windy place. Let it be gone with the wind. Do this once a day.

- ❧ Try to listen to a piece of sad music. It works for some people. In China it's called *"using toxin to attack toxin."* If you feel that this is not your cup of tea, change to a happy type of music.
- ❧ Walk in a flower garden as much as possible. Research shows that having more than 25 percent of green color in your vision will make you much more calm and happier. For the same reason, if you have a garden, spend more time on your garden work.
- ❧ Use a wood comb to gently brush your head from the forehead to the back of your head, from the central to both sides. Use adequate force that is comfortable. The tip of the comb should not be sharp.
- ❧ Treating your feet can moderate your autonomic system, which plays a very important role in your depression.
  - ↳ Soak your feet in hot water (as hot as is comfortable) for 20 minutes every day. If the water reaches your calf, you can get a better result. After soaking, rotate your ankles 20 times (for each foot). Use your hand to rotate each toe clockwise 20 times, then counterclockwise 20 times. Meanwhile repeat silently to yourself, "I am happy now."
  - ↳ Use a hairbrush to tap your soles for five minutes. Pay special attention to the point below the ball of the foot in the center about a third of the distance between the toes and the heel (Ki1). The brush stimulates your soles as a bench of acupuncture needles would (see page 103).
  - ↳ Use an empty, plastic soft drink bottle to pat your bare foot (the top, the sole, and both sides) for three minutes. Keep patting rhythmically about three times per second. About 30 times on each location.
- ❧ Massage your ears: Sit on a chair. Use the thumb and the outside of the index finger to grab your ear and pull in different directions (upwards, downwards, horizontally) for 30 seconds. Grab another location and repeat the same procedure. Meanwhile deeply and slowly inhale and exhale.

Food Therapy

   ☞ Eat nuts with milk:

Ingredients: 2 oz. sesame seeds, 2 oz. walnuts, 1/4 oz. fennel fruits, 50 ml milk, 50 ml sesame oil, 50 ml honey, 2 oz. crystal sugar.

Procedure: Grind walnuts, sesame seeds and fennel into fine powders. Add sugar, honey, sesame oil, and milk. Simmer for 30 minutes on low heat. Store in a jar with lid in the refrigerator. Take 1/4 oz. at a time, three times a day.

Qi Gong

Practice one of the following (whatever you are comfortable with). If you feel it is not right for you, stop the activity.

   ☞ In the morning when the sun has just risen, stand facing the sun in a quiet backyard. Place your feet shoulder width apart. Raise your hands to the sun with the palms up, like you are hugging the sun. Place your tongue against the palate—the area just behind your upper teeth. Breathe naturally. Inhale and visualize the essence of the sun coming down to your palms. Place one hand on the top of your head. Overlap with the other palm. Close your eyes. Image that the essence of the sun pours into your body from the top of your head. Then exhale. Repeat this procedure five times. In Chinese medicine the sun is Yang and the moon is Yin. Depression is the imbalance of Yin and Yang with hyperactivity of Yin. The essence of the sun will help the balance in your body.

   ☞ Do "river of harmonious spirit" exercise. See **Anxiety** section.

Light Therapy

You may also try light therapy, in which you are exposed to intense light from a specially built light box. Research shows that the light may cause some changes in brain's neurochemistry and, therefore, has an antidepressant affect.

Chinese Massage

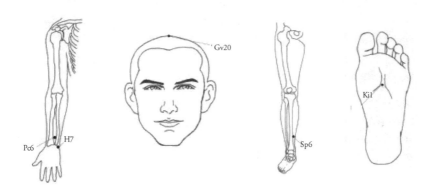

- Place both palms on the chest. Gently push along the ribs to the sides of your body.
- Gently press and knead the following points for one minute:
  - The point two thumb-widths above the wrist crease of the palm side, between the tendons, right under the area where the buckle of the watchstrap would fall (Pc6).
  - The point four finger-widths up from the inside ankle-bone, right behind the leg bone (Sp6).
  - The depression at the meeting point of the wrist crease of the palm side and the line from the little finger (H7).
  - The point located at the center of the top of the head on the line connecting two tips of both ears (Gv20).

Chinese Herbs

- Take the patent herb Xiao Yao Wan. Follow the instructions.

Diabetes

WHAT IS IT AND WHAT CAUSES IT?

It is a disease caused by a malfunction in regulating the blood glucose level. The symptoms are frequent urination, excessive thirst, and fluid intake, and hunger. Type I diabetes is marked by the pancreas making none or little insulin, which is the hormone needed to lower blood glucose levels. Type II diabetes is caused by the inability of the body to use the existing insulin properly. Both can cause high glucose in the blood, and many serious complications will follow.

WHEN SHOULD YOU SEE A DOCTOR?

Mostly cases of diabetes don't show any symptoms at the beginning. If you have a family history of diabetes or have the symptoms previously mentioned, see a doctor. If you have been diagnosed with diabetes, you should always be under a physician's care.

WHAT SHOULD YOU DO IN DAILY LIFE?

- Keep your mood light and optimistic. Research shows psychological factors play a very important role in your health. Every emotional upset will raise your blood sugar.
- You need a diet plan for each meal. You should have a professional work out a special plan for you. You should record the food name and the quantity of your intake, in order to adjust your diet plan according to your blood sugar. Chinese medicine often uses the following foods to help: eel, pumpkin, bitter melon, mung beans, red small beans, Chinese yam, taro root, sesame seeds, walnuts, and onion.
- Exercise is the best medicine to lower your blood sugar. The muscles turn glucose into energy. Walking, swimming, and practicing Qi Gong or Tai Chi are very good activities. Take care not to exercise with an empty stomach.
- Pay more attention to your feet and the shoes you are wearing. See a podiatrist after you have been diagnosed with diabetes.
- Take a warm (not hot) bath.

WHAT SHOULDN'T YOU DO?

- Don't eat snacks. Avoid spicy and heat-inducing foods such as lamb, ginger, hot pepper, cinnamon, or red ginseng. Don't lie down right after a meal.

* Don't over-rest in bed. Being active can help to consume the sugar in your blood.
* Don't put yourself in a stressful situation. Solve the problem before you get angry, which will elevate the adrenaline levels in your blood and increase blood glucose.
* Absolutely no smoking and absolutely no alcohol.
* Avoid any skin damage. For a diabetic, it is very easy to get an infection.
* Do not stop any treatment when your situation gets better.

Folk Remedies

* Use 1 cup of cold water to soak 1/4 oz. of green tea leaves for five hours. Drink frequently. There are substances within the tea leaves that can boost the effect of insulin. These substances lose their effectiveness when boiled.
* Use a toothbrush to slightly brush your soles right below the big bone close to the arch for three minutes, three times a day. Use a spoon to slightly scrub the pad below your thumb, from your wrist crease to the joint of the thumb and the index finger. These areas are the reflex zones of the pancreas.
* Eat pumpkin as main food—about 1 lb. a day for one month.

Food Therapy

* Drink red small bean soup:

    Ingredients: 2 oz. red small beans.

    Procedure: Soak beans in 4 cups water overnight. Put in a pot and bring to a boil. Reduce heat and simmer for an hour. Drink 100 ml. (each time) three times a day for one month.

* Chop a whole onion into eight parts, soak in 500 ml of red wine for 10 days. After it's ready, drink 30 ml before a meal, twice a day.
* Eat millet porridge every morning: Boil 2 oz. of millet with water, then allow it to sit for a while. Skim off the

surface layer. Eat the first half one hour before breakfast. Drink the rest of the porridge during breakfast.

- Steam 4 oz. of fresh Chinese yam. Divide into two portions. Peel and eat twice a day.
- Every morning eat half a box of tofu, cooked any way you prefer.

Qi Gong

Do the three-line relaxing once a day. Repeat the following three times. Take a rest after each cycle.

- Lie down with the tongue tip raised against the hard palate. Slightly close your eyes. Take a deep breath.
- Tell yourself: "Both sides of my head are relaxed, both sides of my neck are relaxed, my two shoulders are relaxed, my upper arms are relaxed, my forearms are relaxed, my wrists are relaxed, my hands are relaxed, my 10 fingers are relaxed."
- Tell yourself: "My face is relaxed, my neck is relaxed, my chest is relaxed, my abdomen is relaxed, my two thighs are relaxed, my knees are relaxed, my two feet are relaxed, my ten toes are relaxed."
- Tell yourself: "The back of my head is relaxed, the back of my neck is relaxed, my back is relaxed, the back of my waist is relaxed, the posterior parts of both thighs are relaxed, the backside of my knees are relaxed, my two calves are relaxed, the two soles of my feet are relaxed."

Chinese Massage

Choose from the following and massage once a day:

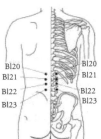
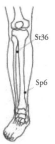
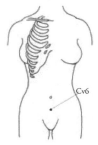

☞ Use your palm to gently push and knead your chest for one minute. Focus on your heart area.

☞ Place your right palm on inside of your left wrist. Scrub up to your armpit for one minute. Change hands to do the other side.

☞ Place your both palms on the upper abdomen. Gently push down, traveling to the lower abdomen for one minute.

☞ Use your palm to gently rub the lower abdomen in a counterclockwise direction, centered at the point two finger-widths below the belly button on the middle of the abdomen for one minute (Cv6).

☞ Use the knuckles to gently press and knead the area on your back two finger-widths on either side of the spine, from the highest point you can reach, down to the point level with the waist, for two minutes (Bl20–Bl23). Change hands to do the other side.

☞ Gently press the depression four finger-widths below the kneecap edge and one thumb-width outside of the shinbone for one minute (St36).

☞ Gently press the point four finger-widths up from the inside anklebone, right behind the leg bone for one minute (Sp6).

Chinese Herbs

☞ Eat pig's pancreas with herbs:

Ingredients: One fresh pig's pancreas (available in some Chinese grocery stores), 2 oz. astragalus root, 3 oz. Chinese pearl barley, 4 oz. Chinese yam.

Procedure: Soak pearl barley in water overnight. Wash and slice the pancreas into small pieces. Slice astragalus into small pieces and wrap with gauze. Place all ingredients in a pot. Add 3 cups of water and bring to a boil. Simmer for another 10 minutes. Discard the astragalus. Add salt and divide into four portions. Eat one portion of the pancreas, yam, and pearl barley a day.

Diarrhea (Chronic)

WHAT IS IT AND WHAT CAUSES IT?

Diarrhea is frequent bowel movements with an unformed, watery stool. It is mainly caused by viral or bacterial infection, intestinal inflammation, lactose intolerance, food poisoning, or some medications.

WHEN SHOULD YOU SEE A DOCTOR?

If you have diarrhea for more than two days, or if the abdominal pain is serious, or if you have bloody or purulent stools, dizziness, or fever, see a doctor.

WHAT SHOULD YOU DO IN DAILY LIFE?

* Drink more water to supply enough fluid to prevent dehydration. Drink lightly brewed green tea. Tea has tannic acid, which may help to control diarrhea.
* If it is caused by food poisoning, skip one or two meals and let the diarrhea run its course. If you have acute diarrhea, eat foods that are easy to digest such as rice soup, noodle soup, soybean milk, egg soup, or chicken broth. Add red dates, Chinese yam, chestnuts, and lotus to your diet.
* Take hot baths. Soak the entire body except your head in hot water for 20 minutes. Do not scald yourself. Do not take a hot bath if you are elderly or a person who has heart problems.
* Do regular exercise such as jogging, walking, or practicing Tai Chi.
* Check your medication to see if it causes diarrhea.

WHAT SHOULDN'T YOU DO?

* Don't use or stop using antibiotics without first consulting your doctor.
* Do not eat greasy or spicy food. Don't eat cold and raw foods, including fruit and salads. Don't eat fried foods.

Avoid alcohol, caffeine, and dairy products except yogurt.

ᵏ Don't sit on damp ground for a long time. Don't expose your abdomen to a cold condition.

Folk Remedies

๛ Eat steamed apples:

Ingredients: Apples.

Procedure: Steam an apple until it becomes soft. Eat one apple three times a day.

๛ Apply salt and green onion:

Ingredients: 1 lb. salt, 1 lb. green onion.

Procedure: Slice green onion into small pieces. Stir-fry them with salt to warm. Place them in a cotton fabric bag. Apply to your belly button and lower abdomen twice a day. Be careful not to burn yourself.

๛ Apply ginger:

Ingredients: Ginger.

Procedure: Crush the ginger into small pieces. Put it on a piece of gauze and apply to your belly button. Use a tape or a bandage to hold it in place. Change every six hours. If you have an allergic skin reaction, discontinue use.

Food Therapy

๛ Eat rice soup with hawthorn fruit:

Ingredients: 1 oz. rice, 1/2 oz. hawthorn fruit, 2 slices ginger, 1/2 oz. sugar.

Procedure: Add ingredients and 3 cups of water to a pot and cook for 20 minutes to make rice soup. Divide into three portions. Drink a portion three times a day for three days.

๛ Eat vinegar and eggs:

Ingredients: 100 ml rice vinegar, 100 ml water, 2 shelled eggs, 1 Tbs. sugar.

Procedure: Put the shelled eggs into vinegar and water to cook until well done. Eat the eggs with the vinegar. Repeat for two days.

☞ Drink burned green tea:

Ingredients: 1 tsp. green tea leaves.

Procedure: Stir-fry the tea leaves in a pan until they become very dark brown. Boil 1 cup of water. Steep the tea leaves for five minutes. Drink twice a day.

☞ Eat brown sugar and liquor:

Ingredients: 1 oz. brown sugar, 50 ml 100-proof vodka.

Procedure: Place the sugar and liquor in a fire-safe bowl. Set on fire and stir continuously with a fire-safe utensil until all sugar is dissolved. (Take great care when burning the sugar. If you feel more comfortable, do this outdoors.) Wait awhile to eat. Repeat for three days.

Chinese Massage

Choose the following and massage once a day:

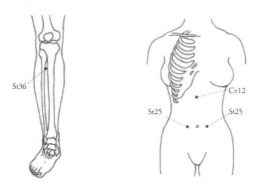

☞ Using your palm, circle and gently press and release around the belly button (navel) from the right lower abdomen up to the right rib, cross the midline to the left rib, and down to the left lower abdomen.

- Using your right palm press and knead the abdomen clockwise for one minute. Using your left palm, gently press and knead the abdomen counterclockwise for one minute.
- Using your thumb, gently press and knead the point halfway between the belly button and the lower edge of the breastbone for two minutes (Cv12).
- Using your thumb, gently press and knead the point two thumb-widths on either side of the belly button (navel) for two minutes (St25).
- Gently press the depression four finger-widths below the kneecap edge and one thumb's-width outside of the shinbone (St36).

Chinese Herbs

- Take the patent herb Shen Ling Bai Zhu Wan. Follow the instructions.
- For the elderly with coldness in abdomen and limbs, diarrhea often happens in early morning. Take the patent herb Jin Gui Shen Qi Wan. Follow the instructions.

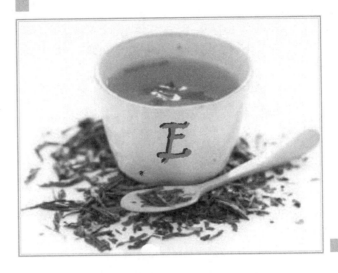

Ear Ringing (Tinnitus)

WHAT IS IT AND WHAT CAUSES IT?

Tinnitus is continuing or intermittent sounds such as ringing, clicking, bussing, hissing, humming, whistling, roaring, or pounding occurring in one or both ears. Tinnitus is caused by inner ear problems or an underlying disease.

WHEN SHOULD YOU SEE A DOCTOR?

Many serious illnesses may cause ear ringing. When this problem has just started, see a doctor immediately.

WHAT SHOULD YOU DO IN DAILY LIFE?

- Taking enough vitamin B, mineral zinc, and magnesium may alleviate the symptoms of tinnitus.
- Stress can make tinnitus worse. Take it easy and relax. Be optimistic about your problems.
- Be aware that some medication may cause tinnitus. Consult with your doctor about the possibilities.

113

WHAT SHOULDN'T YOU DO?

- Don't expose yourself to a noisy environment for a prolonged period.
- Don't drink too much coffee. Stop smoking and avoid alcohol. All these substances can make your tinnitus worse.
- Don't use your finger to dig into your ear. Don't let water stay in your ear.
- Avoid spicy and greasy food.

Folk Remedies

- Use radio or television to mask tinnitus. Listen to music or natural sounds with earphones. Find out ways to distract your attention from your ear ringing.
- Gently pat your ears with your hands 100 times. Do so twice a day.
- Sleep on a pillow with warm salt: Stir-fry salt to moderate warmth. Fill a cotton fabric bag with salt. Lie down on your side so that your ear is resting on the salt bag. Turn to ensure both ears get the treatment. Reheat when it becomes cool. Repeating several times a day may improve the symptoms.
- Use a hairpin or a bundle of toothpicks to gently stimulate the point at the outside edge of the little toe at the corner of the toenail (Bl67) until you have a tingling sensation on the top of your scalp. Repeat several times. Do this once a day.

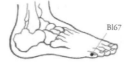

- Clench your teeth on the same side of the infected ear for one minute, two or three times a day. If both ears have problems, clench both sides.

- When you have ear ringing, hold your breath as long as possible. Exhale slowly. Repeat several times. It may help to stop ear ringing.
- Insert Chinese mustard seed powder in the ear:

   Ingredients: Chinese mustard seed (Indian mustard, leaf mustard).

   Procedure: Pound the seeds into fine powder. Wrap them into a small cotton ball. Make sure that no powder can come out the ball. Gently insert the ball into your ear before bedtime. Take it out in the morning. Adjust the size of that cotton ball to fit your ear. Try this for three days. Not for young children.

Food Therapy

- For an acute case, drink chrysanthemum and water chestnut soup:

   Ingredients: 1/2 oz. chrysanthemum flower, 2 oz. water chestnuts. Both are available in Chinese grocery stores.

   Procedure: Place ingredients in a pot, add 3 cups of water, and cook for 10 minutes to make soup. Drink 3 cups once a day for a week.

- For a chronic case eat walnuts: Soak walnuts in salt water for 30 minutes. Take them out and wait for them to dry. Use low heat to stir-fry them until crunchy. Eat 1/2 oz. every morning.

- For a chronic case, drink lotus seed and red date soup:

   Ingredients: 1/2 oz. lotus seeds, 6 red dates, 1/4 oz. pseudostellaria root, 1/2 oz. crystal sugar.

   Procedure: Soak lotus seeds and herb in water overnight. Add water to cover all ingredients and bring to a boil. Reduce heat and simmer for 20 minutes. Discard the pseudostellaria root. Divide into two portions and drink twice a day for a week.

Chinese Massage

Choose from the following and massage once a day:

* Use both your palms to cover the ears. Place your middle finger on top of the index fingers. Use them to gently knock at the back of the head 36 times.
* Use your palms to seal the ears closed, then suddenly open it for 12 times.
* Place your left hand over the head and pull up the right ear 24 times. Change your hands and do the same on the left.
* Use your thumb, index, and middle fingers together to rub the whole ear, from the top to the bottom of the earlobes 36 times.
* Gently press your palms closely against the ears and push up suddenly, then down 36 times.
* Insert your index fingers into your ear and rotate clockwise 12 times. Suddenly pull out. Repeat 12 times.
* Insert your little finger into the ear and pull out 50 times, meanwhile use your upper teeth to knock against the lower teeth 50 times. Use your palms to rub your ears until they become warm.
* Use your index fingers to knead the depression right behind your lower edges of the earlobes 36 times.

Chinese Herbs

* If your ear ringing onsets quickly and sounds like a sea tide or thunderclap, and you have dry throat, bitter mouth, and irritability, take the patent herb Dan Zhi Xiao Yao Wan. Follow the instructions.
* If your ear ringing comes and goes for a prolonged period and is worse at night, take the patent herb Er Long Zuo Ci Wan. Follow the instructions.

Eczema (Atopic Dermatitis)

WHAT IS IT AND WHAT CAUSES IT?

It is a skin inflammation. The red, unbearable itchy skin may be thick, dry, and scaly. Sometimes it can bubble up and ooze. Genetics is the cause for atopic dermatitis.

WHEN SHOULD YOU SEE A DOCTOR?

If you have any kind of skin problem; if you have a bacterial infection such as crusting, oozing, swelling, weeping sores, or a fever; or iof there is no sign of improvement after five days of self-treatment, see a doctor.

WHAT SHOULD YOU DO IN DAILY LIFE?

- Find a trigger such as pollen, chemical solution, or food. Pay special attention to intake of fish, egg, dairy, nuts, and citrus. Be aware that some medications may cause eczema.
- Eat Vitamin B2-rich food such as milk, eggs, Chinese dried mushroom, and green vegetables. Eat more clear-internal-heat-type foods such as mung beans, red small beans, winter melon, cucumber, bitter melon, purslane, or dandelion. Eat more fatty-acid-rich foods such as avocados, salmon, or walnuts.
- Reduce stress as much as possible.
- Exercise regularly to gradually enhance your adjustability to environmental change, and to reduce the allergic risk.

WHAT SHOULDN'T YOU DO?

- Don't scratch the affected area. Don't use hot water to suppress itching. Use a piece of gauze to daub some cold milk onto the infected area. It may give you some relief.
- You probably feel more itching after bathing, drinking alcohol, exposing to sunshine, wearing warm clothes, and mental exertion. You need to avoid these situations as much as possible.

- Don't take too many baths or stay in the bathtub too long. Add 1/2 cup of ground oatmeal to bath water to help relieve itching.
- Avoid overusing soap and cosmetics. Moisturize your skin with heavy cream-based moisturizer.
- Don't wear woolen, silk, or polyester clothes, which will stimulate your skin. Wear loose cotton underwear only.
- Don't eat spicy food such as hot pepper, onion, or garlic. Don't eat lamb, crab, or shrimp. Temporarily eat no high-protein food. No strong tea. Avoid alcohol and coffee.

Folk Remedies

- For oozing eczema, use sliced potato to rub the infected area, three times a day. Peel potato first. Slice into small pieces, or use a blender to make a paste. Apply 1/4-inch thick layer of potato paste to the affected area. Wrap with gauze and clear plastic wrap. Change three times a day. Do not use this treatment if you are allergic to potatoes.
- Grind an aspirin pill to a fine powder. Add water to make a paste. Apply to the affected area twice a day. Do not use this treatment if you are allergic to aspirin.
- In chronic cases, use a juicer to make water spinach (also called hollow vegetable, available in Chinese grocery stores) and celery juice. Mix them together. Apply the mixture to the affected area. Do not use this treatment if you are allergic to spinach and/or celery.

Food Therapy

- Eat four apricots a day for three days. Also, apply apricot meat to the affected area.
- Drink red bean soup for an acute case:

    Ingredients: 1/2 oz. red small beans, 1/2 oz. corn silk, 1 oz. Chinese pearl barley.

    Procedure: Soak beans and pearl barley in water overnight. Wrap corn silk with gauze and put it in a pot.

Add other ingredients to the pot with 3 cups of water and bring to a boil. Reduce heat and simmer until beans are soft. Eat pearl barley and beans, and drink the soup once a day for one week.

Chinese Herbs

☞ Drink mung bean and kelp soup with herb for an acute case:

Ingredients: 1 oz. mung beans, 1 oz. kelp (dried seaweed), 1/2 oz. houttuynia, sugar.

Procedure: Soak mung beans and kelp in water overnight. Wrap the herb in gauze and place all ingredients in a pot. Add 4 cups of water and bring to a boil. Reduce heat and simmer until beans are soft. Discard the herb. Eat mung beans and kelp, and drink soup once a day for a week.

☞ Drink fruit soup for a chronic case:

Ingredients: 1 oz. mulberry, 1 oz. lily bulb, 10 dates, 1/4 oz. olive.

Procedure: Add ingredients to 4 cups of water and bring to a boil. Reduce heat and simmer for 20 minutes. Divide into two portions. Eat twice a day for a week.

Eyestrain

WHAT IS IT AND WHAT CAUSES IT?

It is blurred vision, red or dry eyes, and a heavy sensation in the eyelids caused by the overuse of your eyes.

WHEN SHOULD YOU SEE A DOCTOR?

If you have uncomfortable eyes constantly, double vision, or dizziness, see a doctor.

WHAT SHOULD YOU DO IN DAILY LIFE?

☀ Let your eyes rest by looking far away for five minutes every hour.

* Adjust your computer monitor's contrast to make reading more comfortable. Use a big font if possible.
* Do eye exercises:
  + Close your eyes for five seconds. Quickly open it. Repeat this procedure several times.
  + Close your eyes. Move your eyeballs clockwise five times. Move them counterclockwise five times.
  + Use the thumb-side edges of both palms to gently press and knead the area from the frame of eyes, to the temple, above the ears, and to the back of your head.

Folk Remedies

* Using your thumb, index, and middle fingers to pull down your ears 30 times.
* Sit on a chair and close your eyes. Rub both of your hands until you feel warm. Lightly cover your eyes with your hands for 30 seconds. Meanwhile, imagine that two light beams are coming into your eyes. Repeat this procedure five times. Slowly open your eyes and look at the horizon for a while.
* Apply a sliced cucumber over your eyes for 10 minutes.

Food Therapy

* Drink chrysanthemum flower tea:

    Ingredients: 1/4 oz. chrysanthemum flower, available in Chinese grocery stores.

    Procedure: Steep flower with boiled water. Cover and wait for 10 minutes. Drink once a day for three days.
* Eat black bean with lycium fruit:

    Ingredients: 10 oz. black beans, 1 oz. lycium fruit, 1 Tbs. sugar

    Procedure: Soak beans in water overnight. Add enough water to cover the beans in a pot. Bring to a boil. Simmer it until beans are soft. Add sugar and lycium fruits. Simmer for another five minutes. Store in a jar. Take 1 Tbs. at a time, twice a day for a week.

Chinese Massage

Choose the following and massage each point for 30 seconds or one minute once a day.

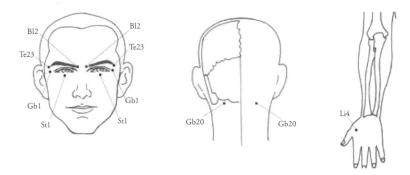

🌿 Knead the point just under the pupil of your eye, in the middle of the ridge of the eye socket (St1).

🌿 Knead the point in the depression, half a finger's width outside the corner of the eye (Gb1).

🌿 Knead the depression at the outer edge of the eyebrow (Te23).

🌿 Knead the central point on the eyebrow, and the temples.

🌿 Knead the depression on the beginning of the eyebrow (Bl2).

🌿 Close your eyes. Use your middle fingers to knead the depression between the eyebrows and eyeballs, meanwhile using your thumb to knead the both temples.

🌿 Press and knead the depression at the bottom of the skull, outside of the two big muscles on the neck, which you can feel by bending your head down, neck forward (Gb20).

🌿 With your thumb against the index finger, use your other thumb to press the webbing where it bulges up the highest (Li4).

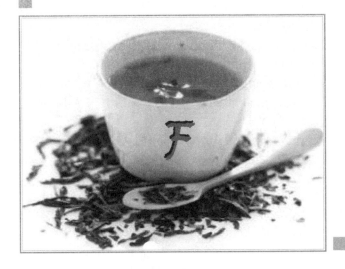

Fatigue

WHAT IS IT AND WHAT CAUSES IT?

It is the feeling of exhaustion and low energy. Everyone has felt fatigued once in a while and, indeed, it sometimes is a normal part of life. But there are people who are more prone to fatigue. No matter what they do, they feel tired and groggy all the time.

WHEN SHOULD YOU SEE A DOCTOR?

See a doctor if your fatigue lasts too long or is accompanied by other symptoms. Fatigue may be related to many serious diseases such as diabetes, hepatitis, or thyroid problems.

WHAT SHOULD YOU DO IN DAILY LIFE?

* Sleep is a crucial factor in fatigue. Maintain a regular sleep schedule and don't sleep too little or too much.

- Adequate nutrition is also necessary to maintain energy. Make sure to eat full meals of all food groups, especially a good breakfast. Take multivitamins daily.
- Schedule your work and activities sensibly so you don't get overloaded.
- Drink plenty of water to avoid dehydration, which can lead to fatigue.
- Keep correct posture at work or rest, no matter whether you are sitting, standing, or laying down, it will make you much more relaxed.
- After coming off a stressful and intense period, reward yourself with something relaxing and enjoyable such as a massage or a vacation.
- Exercise will produce energy. Here are some simple things you can do: Take a fast walk for 20 to 30 minutes a day. Practicing Tai Chi can both energize the body and sooth your mind.
- Take a hot shower. Let the warm water hit the top of your head for three minutes. Meanwhile keep your mind blank. The elderly or someone with a heart problem should not do this.
- Sing out loud twice a day, preferably in the outdoors where you can deeply breath in fresh air. This will increase your oxygen intake and improve your circulation.
- Social and psychological factors play an important role in fatigue. If you have such a problem, deal with it first.

WHAT SHOULDN'T YOU DO?

- Don't smoke or drink alcohol.

Folk Remedies

- During working hours, you can do the following exercises:
  - Stand in front of a wall with your back facing it and your heels about 5 inches away. Backward, gently hit the wall with your back. Do so 10 times. Make sure the wall is smooth.

- ⇝ Raise your shoulders up towards your ears and lower them. Repeat 10 times.
- ⇝ Use your palms to hold a golf ball. Continuously rotate it for three minutes to stimulate the center of each palm.
- ⇝ Put two golf balls on the floor under your feet and roll them around with your soles for three minutes.

- ☞ Rub some Chinese Tiger Balm on both temples. The smell of the balm will reinvigorate you. If you have an allergic reaction, discontinue use.

Food Therapy

- ☞ Eat cooked bananas:

  Ingredients: 1 ripe banana.

  Procedure: Peel banana. Cut into pieces. Place them in a pan with 1 cup of water. Bring to boil. Simmer for five minutes. Eat one banana a day for a prolonged period.

- ☞ Drink herb wine:

  Ingredients: 250 ml rice wine, 1/2 oz. white ginseng, 1/2 oz. lycium fruit.

  Procedure: Chop the ginseng into slices. Mix with lycium fruit. Soak them in wine for seven days. Shake the concoction several times a day. Drink 15 ml morning and night for a week.

- ☞ Drink ginger milk: Cook 150 ml milk with 1 slice of ginger for two minutes on low heat. Drink at breakfast.

- ☞ Eat chicken with herbs:

  Ingredients: One whole chicken, 1/4 oz. astragalus root, 1/2 oz. Chinese yam, 1/4 oz. codonopsis, 1/4 oz. dang gui, green onions, ginger, and other seasonings if desired.

  Procedure: Wrap all herbs with gauze. Add adequate water to chicken to last until the chicken is well done.

Divide into three portions. Eat the meat and drink the
soup once a day for three days.

Chinese Massage

Choose any combination of the following you are comfortable
with and gently press and knead each point for one or two minutes
once a day:

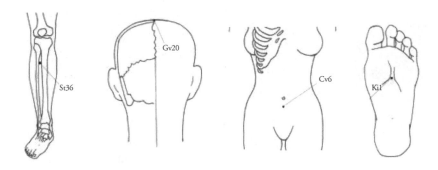

- ≈ The point below the ball of the foot in the center, about
  1/3 of the distance between the toes and the heel (Ki1).
- ≈ The point two finger-widths below the belly button (navel) on the middle of the abdomen (Cv6)
- ≈ The center on the top of your head on the line connecting the two tips of your ears. (Gb20).
- ≈ The depression four finger-widths below the kneecap edge
  and one thumb's-width outside of the shinbone (St36).

Qi Gong

- ≈ Regulate the body:
  - ⊱ Use your palm to pat your whole body as follows: from
    the upper arm to the forearm, from your shoulder to
    the chest, and abdomen, from the lower back to the
    buttock, and from the thigh down to the calf. Use your
    fingers to gently press against the scalp along the
    centerline, starting from the front and working to the
    back of the head for two minutes. Then gently tap
    against the scalp with your palms for one minute.

- ⊢ Use all your fingers to gently grasp your scalp. Use your thumb, index, and middle fingers to grasp the muscles on the back on your neck.
- ⊢ Use your palms to dry wash your face. Sitting with closed eyes, rub your hands together until warm. Use four fingers to gently wipe your face from your forehead to both sides of the nose, to the lips, to the lower jaw, to underneath the ears, and up to the temples. Repeat nine times, then repeat in the opposite direction.

- ☞ Regulate the breath:
  - ⊢ Stretch your arms and chest nine times.
  - ⊢ Yawn vigorously nine times.
  - ⊢ Deeply inhale and exhale nine times.

- ☞ Regulate the mind: Rub your hands against each other until they are warm. If you are male, place the left palm on the lower abdomen, and overlap your right palm. Gently and slowly rub and knead nine times counterclockwise, then clockwise nine times. Meanwhile silently repeat any simple sentence, that is important to you, such as "Fatigue is gone." If you are female, do the same, except place your right palm on the lower abdomen and overlap with the left palm.

Chinese Herbs

- ☞ If you have tiredness with irritability, depression, or insomnia, take the patent herb Xiao Yao Wan. Follow the instructions.
- ☞ If you have tiredness with weak knees, an aversion to cold, and lowered sexual desire, take the patent herb Jin Gui Shen Qi Wan. Follow the instructions.
- ☞ If you are recovering from a surgery or serious disease, and are dizzy, have shortness of breath, or a pale complexion, take the patent herb Shi Quan Da Bu Wan. Follow the instructions.
- ☞ If you are tired with a poor appetite, loose stool, and feel drowsy, take the patent herb Xiang Sha Yang Wei Wan. Follow the instructions.

Fibromyalgia

WHAT IS IT AND WHAT CAUSES IT?

Fibromyalgia is characterized by pain and stiffness in the muscles, ligaments, tendons, and fibers. The pain gets worse with pressure on many specific spots. It is also accompanied with profound fatigue, weakness, and sleep disorder. The symptoms are weather related and worsen in cold or damp conditions, or by physical overexertion. The cause of fibromyalgia is still unknown.

WHEN SHOULD YOU SEE A DOCTOR?

If you have constant muscle pain and sleep disorder, see a doctor.

WHAT SHOULD YOU DO IN DAILY LIFE?

- Try to get an adequate amount of sleep. Refer to the **Insomnia** section. Sleep on a hard mattress.
- Take a hot bath with Epsom salts every morning or evening. Follow the instructions.
- Apply a warm, wet towel to the area in pain and cover with clear plastic wrap. Then apply a heating pad over it for 15 minutes.
- Drink plenty of water or vegetable juice to flush out toxins.
- Exercise regularly: walk, swim, or practice Tai Chi. You may feel more pain at the beginning, but if you gradually increase the workout and persist for a couple of months, it will significantly ease the pain of fibromyalgia.

WHAT SHOULDN'T YOU DO?

- Don't eat fried foods. Avoid caffeine and alcohol. Don't eat too many sweets.

Folk Remedies

- Apply warm salt: Stir-fry 1 lb. of salt until warm. Wrap in three layers of gauze and apply to the painful spot for 15 minutes, twice a day. Take care not to burn yourself.
- Apply tofu with vinegar:
  - Ingredients: Tofu, rice vinegar.
  - Procedure: Cut a 1/4-inch slice of tofu and use a fork to punch a lot of holes. Soak it in a bowl with vinegar. Use a microwave to warm the tofu and apply to the painful area for 20 minutes. Reheat the tofu if necessary. If you have an allergic skin reaction, discontinue use.
- Working on your feet to move your Qi and improve blood circulation:
  - Walk on gravel: Build a 2-foot wide, 20-foot long path with smooth gravel on flat ground. Walk barefoot for 15 to 20 minutes a day for a prolonged period. At the beginning, you can wear a pair of socks to reduce the uncomfortable feeling. If your ankles feel tired, stop doing this.
  - When you are watching TV, place several golf balls in a box and move these balls around with the soles of your feet as long as possible.
  - Walk with the front part of your feet (lifting the heel) at home.
  - Place a baseball bat or a pipe of 1 1/2 or 2 inches diameter on the floor. Slowly roll it back and forth with your soles for 20 minutes a day.
- Massage with a low-power vacuum cleaner: Take the head or brush away. Use the opening of the pipe to suck your painful spot. Lightly lift the pipe, but don't leave the skin. Hold for 10 seconds, then move to another spot.

Food Therapy

☞ Drink pearl barley soup with herb:

Ingredients: 1 oz. Chinese pearl barley, 1/4 oz. siler.

Procedure: Wrap the herbs with gauze. Add herbs and 2 cups of water to a pot and bring to a boil. Reduce heat and simmer for 20 minutes. Discard the herbs. Drink the decoction once a day for a week.

☞ Drink ginger with brown sugar:

Ingredients: 2 slices ginger, 1 Tbs. brown sugar.

Procedure: Brew with boiled water and drink for a week.

Chinese Massage

Don't massage the painful spot directly. Lie down on your stomach. Ask a family member to do any combination of the following you are comfortable with and massage once a day:

☞ Use four fingers *gently* to press and knead the back for two minutes to warm the muscles. Use the heel of the palm to *gently* push the area on both sides of the spine three times to loosen the muscles.

☞ Stand on one side. Use the index, middle, and ring fingers to *gently* rub the muscles two finger-widths beside the spine from the upper back down to the waist. Repeat three times. Move to the other side and do the same.

☞ Use the thumb, index, and middle fingers to *gently* grasp the painful muscles and tendons, squeezing, lifting, and releasing *quickly* for three times.

☞ Find the most painful point first. Use the thumb to *gently* flick the painful muscles and tendons in perpendicular direction to the muscles three times.

Refer to other sections, which may be related to your pain.

Chinese Herbs

☞ Take the patent herb Vine Essence Pill. Follow the instructions.

Frostbite

WHAT IS IT AND WHAT CAUSES IT?

Frostbite is damage to the skin and underlying tissue caused by exposure to extreme cold for a prolonged period. It starts with a "pins and needles" sensation, followed by numbness. The skin will become red and painful. In severe cases there are blisters with red or even purple color. In most cases it happens on the hands, feet, nose, and ears.

WHEN SHOULD YOU SEE A DOCTOR?

If you have severe frostbite, you need to see a doctor.

WHAT SHOULD YOU DO IN DAILY LIFE?

↣ Wear warm and loose clothing and shoes to get better local blood circulation.

↣ In the early stage (no open blister) soak your hands or feet in a paraffin bathtub (available in a department store) once a day. Follow the instructions. Afterward, apply 100-percent aloe vera gel to the affected area.

↣ In an early stage, you can place your hands or feet under a light bulb for 20 minutes. Keep it a distance away, as long as it feels warm and comfortable, twice a day. Afterward, apply 100-percent aloe vera gel to the affected area.

WHAT SHOULDN'T YOU DO?

↣ Don't rub with snow or soak in cold water. Don't use hot water to warm the affected area. Don't use fire to warm the affected area.

↣ If it itches, don't scratch the affected area.

Folk Remedies

- Apply cherries: First take the seeds out. If the affected area is not too big, apply cherries directly on the affected spot. Otherwise, pound several cherries first, wrap in gauze, and apply to the affected area for three to five hours a day. You can also rub the area with cherry wine:

  Ingredients: 8 oz. cherries (best if not totally ripe; if fresh cherries are not available, use canned), 500 ml 80-proof vodka.

  Procedure: Soak cherries in the vodka for seven days. Use a cotton ball to apply mixture to the affected area five times a day.

- Wash with black peppercorns: Grind 1/4 oz. black peppercorns. Add peppercorns to 1 cup of water and bring to a boil. Wash the affected area while it is still warm, two or three times a day. If you have an allergic reaction, discontinue use.

- Apply cactus: Remove the needles from the cactus first and then pound it into a paste. Apply to the affected area. Wrap with gauze. Change once a day.

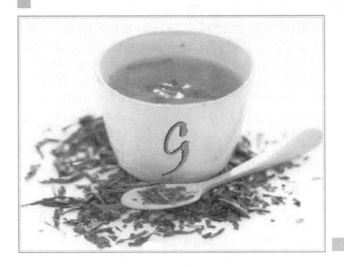

Gout

WHAT IS IT AND WHAT CAUSES IT?

Gout is joint inflammation caused by heightened uric acid levels in the blood. It deposits on the joints, and causes inflammation. The symptoms are sudden pain in a joint (often the big toe) with redness, swelling, and fever. Eating too much food with high purines, having kidney problems, and taking certain medications can elevate blood levels of uric acid. It can also be genetic.

WHEN SHOULD YOU SEE A DOCTOR?

If you have sudden swelling and pain in a joint, see a doctor.

WHAT SHOULD YOU DO IN DAILY LIFE?

* When you have an attack, rest and raise the painful limb. Apply a cold pack for 20 minutes three times a day. It reduces the swelling and pain.

> ✻ Drink at least 8 cups of water and juice a day to flush out excess uric acid.
>
> ✻ Eat less acidic foods. Eat more alkaline foods such as kelp, Chinese cabbage, cucumber, celery, eggplant, daikon radish, tomatoes, onion, apples, bananas, peaches, and pears. Eat more fresh or canned cherries, cherry juice, or strawberries. These basic foods will neutralize the uric acid.
>
> ✻ If you are overweight, controlling your weight is key. Heavier people have a tendency to have a high level of uric acid.

WHAT SHOULDN'T YOU DO?

> ✻ Avoid purine-rich foods such as animal organs, fatty meats, mussels, sardines, caviar, crab, and anchovies. Limit the intake of spinach, dry beans, mushroom, cauliflower, and asparagus in your diet.
>
> ✻ Don't eat too much at a time. Reduce salt intake. Avoid spicy food, strong condiments, or MSG.
>
> ✻ Avoid alcohol and beer—alcohol will increase uric acid levels.

Folk Remedies

> ☙ Take aloe vera juice orally, or apply the gel to painful spots.
>
> ☙ If gout chronically occurs in the foot, soak your feet in hot water with charcoal:
>
>> **Ingredients:** 8 oz. charcoal.
>>
>> **Procedure:** Boil the charcoal in hot water for 10 minutes. Remove the charcoal and wait for it to dry. Put charcoal in a cotton fabric bag and place the bag in a container. Gradually pour warm water into this container and soak your feet for 30 minutes, once a day for one month. Be careful, as the charcoal stains. You can dry the charcoal and reuse.

Food Therapy

☞ Drink pearl barley and rice soup with mung beans:

Ingredients: 1 oz. Chinese pearl barley, 1/2 oz. mung beans, 2 oz. rice.

Procedure: Soak beans in water overnight. Add beans and 4 cups of water to a pot and bring to a boil. Reduce heat and simmer until beans are soft. Drink twice a day.

☞ Eat 1 Tbs. of blackberry juice and 1 Tbs. of strawberry juice, three times a day.

Chinese Massage

☞ Use the thumb to push the joint that is in pain and its surrounding area for two minutes.

☞ Use the thumb to press and knead the spot that is in pain and its surrounding area for two minutes.

Chinese Herbs

☞ Take the patent herb Du Huo Ji Sheng Wan. Follow the instructions.

Groin Strain (Groin Pull)

WHAT IS IT AND WHAT CAUSES IT?

Groin strain is adductor muscle injuries caused by overexertion. The symptoms are a sharp pain or tenderness in the upper inner thigh, that gets worse with activities.

WHEN SHOULD YOU SEE A DOCTOR?

If the pain bothers your daily activities, or if you have no sign of improvement two days after self-treatment, see a doctor.

WHAT SHOULD YOU DO IN DAILY LIFE?

» In acute cases stop your activity right away. Apply ice for 15 to 20 minutes on the injured thigh several times a day. Loosely wrap the injured thigh with an elastic bandage.

WHAT SHOULDN'T YOU DO?

» Don't use any heat at the very beginning because it is very hard to tell if there is inside bleeding.

Folk Remedies

☞ Apply tofu with vinegar:

Ingredients: Tofu, rice vinegar.

Procedure: Cut a 1/4-inch slice of tofu and use a fork to punch a lot of holes. In acute cases freeze the tofu in a refrigerator for five minutes. Soak it in a bowl with vinegar. Apply the tofu to the painful area for 20 minutes. In chronic cases, use a microwave to warm the tofu and apply to the painful area for 20 minutes. Reheat the tofu if necessary. If you have an allergic skin reaction, discontinue use.

☞ In a chronic case, cook 1 oz. of green tea leaves: Apply the warm tea leaves to the painful spots. In an acute case, wait until the leaves cool, then apply to the painful spots.

☞ In chronic cases, massage with a low-power vacuum cleaner: Take the head or brush away. Use the opening of the pipe to suck at your thigh. Lightly lift the pipe, but don't lose contact with the skin. Hold for 10 seconds, then move to another spot.

Chinese Massage

Do not massage in acute cases.

☞ Use the heel of your palm to gently press and knead the inner thigh from the top of your leg to your knee for two minutes.

- Gently press and knead the painful point in the top of your injured thigh for two minutes.

- Use the thumb and other fingers to grasp the muscles of your inner thigh from the top of your injured leg down to the knee joint for two minutes.

- Use your thumb to gently press and knead the following points for one minute:

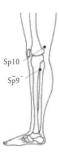

- The point right in the depression inside of the calf under the knee, behind the leg bone (Sp9).

- The point on the top of inside edge of the knee. Flex your knee and place your hand on the kneecap. The point is where your thumb touches (Sp10).

Chinese Herbs

- Take the patent herb Yu Nan Bai Yao. Follow the instructions.

- Apply the patent herb tincture Zheng Gu Shui to the painful spot. Follow the instructions. If you have an allergic reaction, discontinue use.

- Apply the herb patch Shang Shi Zhi Tong Gao. If you have an allergic reaction, discontinue use.

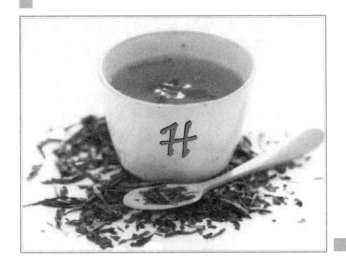

Hair Loss

WHAT IS IT AND WHAT CAUSES IT?

Normally an old hair falls out, a new one grows in. But if the old one is gone and the new one doesn't come out, you have a hair loss problem. The male pattern of hair loss is marked by a receding hair-line at the temples and thinning hair on the top of the head. Female pattern is thinning all over. Alopecia areata is another type marked by hair loss in coin-like patches. There are many causes such as aging, poor nutrition, genetics, some medications, stress, or disease. Hair loss can also be caused by anorexia because the body doesn't get enough fat to keep the hair follicles healthy.

WHEN SHOULD YOU SEE A DOCTOR?

If you suddenly lose hair, see a doctor.

WHAT SHOULD YOU DO IN DAILY LIFE?

- ⋇ Use baby shampoo. Comb gently.

- Eat iron-rich foods such as lean red meat, soybeans, black beans, eggs, fish, shrimp, spinach, carrots, potatoes, and bananas. Some women lose hair because they have a lack of iron in their bodies. Increase the intake of iodide found in foods such as seaweed and oysters. Drink more meat bone soup.
- Increase the intake of vegetable protein such as corn, black sesame seeds, and soybeans. Eat more basic food such as fresh vegetables and fruits.
- Take enough Vitamin complex every day.
- Reduce stress, as it may cause hair loss.

Folk Remedies

- Wash hair with vinegar: Mix 200 ml rice vinegar with 1,000 ml warm water. Wash your hair while it is still warm. Use clear warm water to rinse. Do this twice a week for a prolonged period, or you can wash hair with a soupspoon of soybean milk and 1 Tbs. of vinegar every other day for a prolonged period. Do skin test first. If there is an allergic reaction, discontinue use.
- Wash hair with salt water: Put 2 oz. of salt in a basin half full of water. Soak hair. Knead and rub your hair for two or three minutes. Then shampoo hair and rinse in warmed salt water again. Rinse with plain water two times. Do this twice a week for a prolonged period.
- Rub liquor with oriental arborvitae leaves:

  Ingredients: Fresh oriental arborvitae leaves, 80-proof vodka.

  Procedure: Soak leaves in vodka in a sealed bottle for one week. Remove the leaves. Use a cotton swab to dab the liquor on your head two times a day for a prolonged period. Do skin test first, if there is an allergic reaction, stop.

Food Therapy

- Eat 1/2 oz. of sunflower seeds every day.
- Soak five red dates in water until puffy. Cook the dates

with 1 1/2 cups of water in a pot for 10 minutes. Crash the egg into the pot and cook for another 30 seconds. Eat before bedtime.

☞ Eat sesame seeds and walnuts with sugar:

Ingredients: 8 oz. black sesame seed, 8 oz. walnuts, 2 oz. sugar.

Procedure: Stir-fry sesame seeds and walnuts until well done. Don't overcook. Place sugar in a pan with a little water. Heat and mix to make a thick sauce. Add sesame seeds and walnuts. Stir well. Turn off the heat. Pour onto a big plate with a little cooking oil on the surface. Eat 2 oz. at a time, twice a day.

Chinese Massage

☞ Use your fingers to comb through your hair 60 times, twice a day.

☞ Use both of your hands to hold both sides of the head and gently push the skin on the scalp towards the top of your head 60 times, twice a day.

☞ Use your index and third fingers to rub and knead your head. Move your fingers continuously, as if drawing a small circle, from the forehead to the top, down to the back of the head. Then start from the forehead to the temple down to the back of the head. Each round lasts one or two minutes.

Chinese Herbs

☞ Drink fleece flower root tea:

Ingredients: 1/2 oz. processed fleece flower root.

Procedure: Cut the fleece flower root into small pieces. Soak in a coffee maker with boiled water for four to eight hours until the color becomes brownish red. Drink as tea. Add more boiled water into the coffee maker, until the color of the tea becomes light. Meanwhile, use a magnet to rub the affected area.

Hangovers

WHAT IS IT AND WHAT CAUSES IT?

The symptoms of hangovers are headaches, dry mouth, nausea, or vomiting. Usually it takes a day to fade away, but here are some methods to alleviate the symptoms.

WHEN SHOULD YOU SEE A DOCTOR?

If your symptoms are serious or you don't feel better after 24 hours, you should see a doctor. Alcohol poisoning can be fatal.

WHAT SHOULD YOU DO IN DAILY LIFE?

- If you know ahead of time that you will be drinking alcohol, drink 1 cup of cabbage juice first to protect you.
- Drinking a lot of water will moderate the effect of alcohol, especially before going to bed. Keep a glass of water on the nightstand.
- Eat some tomatoes, oranges, apples, pears, or watermelon. The fructose contained in these fruits and vegetables can help process alcohol. You could also drink fruit juice.

WHAT SHOULDN'T YOU DO?

- Don't drink on an empty stomach.
- Don't believe in the old saying that drinking tea after consuming alcohol will relieve your hangover. Caffeine can make you even more dehydrated.
- Don't drink more alcohol to treat hangover symptoms. This will only make it worse.
- Don't stay in bed constantly. If you are capable of being active, get up and walk around.
- Don't hold back your vomiting. It will flush unabsorbed alcohol from your body.

Folk Remedies

☙ Mix 4 Tbs. of rice vinegar, 1 Tbs. of brown sugar, and two slices of raw ginger in 2 cups of water. Boil the mixture and drink.

☙ Use a juicer to make juice from 1 lb. of daikon radish. Add 1 Tbs. of vinegar to drink.

☙ Crush 3 oz. of mung beans in a blender. Cook 5 cups of water with bean powder on low heat for 30 minutes. Drink a cup of the concoction every hour.

☙ Taking a Vitamin B-50 pill can lower the effects of hangovers.

☙ Use a wood comb gently to tap the vertex of your head for three minutes. Use adequate force. The tip of the comb should not be sharp. Then use the comb to gently tap both soles of your feet for three minutes. The comb works like acupuncture needles.

Chinese Massage

☙ Gently press and knead the point four finger-widths up from the inside anklebone, right behind the leg bone for two minutes (Sp6).

☙ Gently press and knead the depression at the meeting point of the wrist crease of the palm side and the line from the little finger for two minutes (H7).

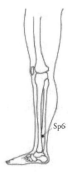
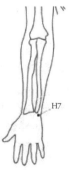

Headaches (Chronic)

WHAT IS IT AND WHAT CAUSES IT?

There are three kinds of chronic headaches, other than those caused by underlying diseases:

- *Tension headache* is marked by a dull, steady pressure kind of pain, which can be in any part of your head, or throughout your head, or the back of your head. It is mostly caused by muscle contraction.
- *Migraine headache* is characterized by throbbing, pulsating pain,mostly on one side. It is sometimes accompanied with nausea, vomiting, and dizziness. The cause often is the head blood vessels expanding and constricting.
- *Cluster headache* is marked by severe, steady pain around or behind one eye.

Science does not completely understand the reason for headaches yet. Stress, depression, lack of sleep, a specific food allergy, and even sexual intercourse may all cause headaches. The triggering factor and modes of relief vary from person to person.

WHEN SHOULD YOU SEE A DOCTOR?

If you have the following types of headaches, you need to see a doctor: Sudden onset with fever and neck stiffness, or frequent headaches with increasing intensity, accompanied with dizziness, numbness, blurred vision, and pain in different locations, or other medical problems coming along with headaches.

WHAT SHOULD YOU DO IN DAILY LIFE?

- Try to find the triggering factors by keeping a diary, which could reveal activity, food, or medication that is associated with your headaches.

- Take a hot shower or run cold water over your head to see if heat or cold helps. If so, buy a reusable gel pack and apply it to your forehead or the back of your neck. Soak your hands in cold water for as long as you can or soak your hands in warm water for as long as you can. Add hot water continuously to regulate the temperature. Repeat several times a day.
- Apply Tiger Balm or lavender oil to the forehead and the temple.
- A cup of strong black tea or coffee may provide some relief. Note that for some people drinking coffee may actually cause a headache. Drinking 1 cup of hot water with 1 tsp. of ginger powder may help, too.
- Use music to distract your attention from your headache. Place one hand on the volume control of a CD player. Close your eyes and listen to your favorite music. Move your hand or foot to the rhythm. When your pain becomes stronger, turn up the volume. When you feel less pain, turn the volume down. Your mind is always on the music, not on the pain.
- Try humor therapy. Watch comedy shows as much as possible. Laughter is the best medicine for tension headaches.
- Exercise regularly. Practicing Tai Chi is a very good choice for healing headaches.
- Enough sleep helps to relieve tension and migraine headaches.

WHAT SHOULDN'T YOU DO?

- The first time you have a headache, don't take painkillers before a medical examination, because they will make it more difficult to diagnose the problem.
- Do not smoke. Do not drink alcohol.
- Don't eat too much salty food—sodium makes blood vessels constrict, which can cause a headache. Don't eat

too much or too little at each meal. Eat more vegetables and fruits. Don't eat fatty and spicy foods. For migraines, avoid hot dogs, ham, sausage, aged cheese, MSG, nuts, peanuts, and chocolate. Drink less coffee if you are a heavy coffee drinker.

* When you catch cold or flu, rest and don't use your brain too much.

* Avoid placing yourself in stressful situations. Irritation and nervousness will make your headache worse.

Folk Remedies

* Besides aerobic exercise, you can do the following exercises to get relief:

    * Stretch your neck: Place your right index finger on the left chin and the right thumb on the lower jaw. Slowly turn your head to the right and look back. Stretch the left arm to cross over the top of your head and touch the top of the right ear. Slowly turn down your head toward your chest. After 10 seconds, return to a normal position. Switch your hands and do the same on the other side. If you feel dizzy, stop. Repeat for three cycles, two times a day.

    * Breathing with abdomen: Look at a fixed object. Inhale through your nose by inflating your abdomen. Exhale through the mouth by constricting the abdomen.

    * Pulling both earlobes gently 50 times with your thumb and index finger may relieve pain in your temple.

* Before you go to bed, fill two tubs: one with warm water and one with cold water. Alternately soak your feet in each for three minutes. Repeat several times.

* Soak your hands in hot water (as hot as is comfortable) for 30 minutes. Add more hot water to maintain the temperature. Repeat three times a day.

🍃 Roll an unbroken boiled egg (while it is still hot and comfortable for your skin) on the painful spot of your head. Sometimes this kind of massage will relieve your tension headache right away.

Food Therapy

🍃 If you have an aversion to cold, drink green tea with ginger and sugar:

Ingredients: 1/8 oz. green tea leaves, 1/2 oz. brown sugar, 1/4 oz. ginger.

Procedure: Brew the ingredients with boiled water. Drink as tea.

🍃 If you have an aversion to heat, drink mung beans and rice soup:

Ingredients: 2 oz. mung beans, 2 oz. rice.

Procedure: Soak mung beans in water overnight. Add 3 cups of water, rice, and beans to a pot, cook to make rice soup. Drink two times a day for three days.

Qi Gong

Do the following step by step:

🍃 Lie down comfortably in a quiet room and take several deep breaths. Close your eyes and breathe naturally.

🍃 Tell yourself, "My head is relaxed, my face is relaxed, my neck is relaxed, my shoulders are relaxed, my arms are relaxed, my hands are relaxed, my fingers are relaxed, my chest is relaxed, my abdomen is relaxed, my legs are relaxed, my feet are relaxed, my toes are relaxed, my whole body is totally relaxed."

🍃 Imagine a river flowing from the top center of your head down to your chest, stomach, and abdomen. The river then divides into two streams flowing into each leg and comes out the soles of your feet. It flows away from you, flows on, flows on, becomes smaller and smaller, and finally disappears. Meanwhile, think of your pain flowing along with this creek, leaving you forever. Repeat this visualization once a day.

Chinese Massage

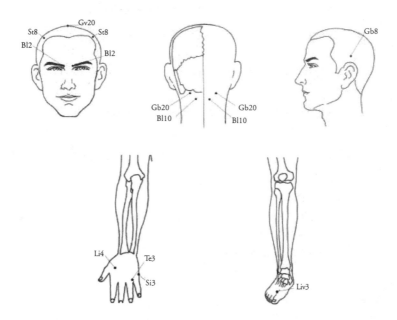

- Comb your hair and scalp with your fingertips. Brush your hair gently from the forehead to the back of the neck. Brush your hair gently from the top to both sides of the head. Apply pressure gradually from light to slightly heavy, until your scalp becomes warm.

- Gently press and knead the point in the depression at the bottom of the skull, outside of the two big muscles on the neck, which you can feel by bending down your neck (Gb20).

- Use the outer edge of your little finger to knock every joint between adjacent fingers of other hand. Change hands to do the other side.

- For pain in the side of the head, add the following:

- ☞ Use the pad of your thumb to gently press, wipe, and knead both temples. Push toward to the area above your ears (Gb8).
- ☞ Gently press and knead the point between the ring and little fingers in the depression right below the two knuckles on the back of the hand (Te3).

☞ For pain in front of the head, add the following:
- ☞ Gently press and knead the depression on the beginning of the eyebrow (Bl2).
- ☞ With your thumb against the index finger; use your other hand to pinch and gently press the webbing where it bulges up the highest (Li4).

☞ For pain in back of the head, add the following:
- ☞ Gently press and knead the point on the nape of the neck, just inside the hairline, two finger-widths on either side of the spine in the depression on the side of the large neck muscle (Bl10).
- ☞ Make a slight fist. Gently press and knead the point on the side of your hand, just below the little finger joint at the end of the crease (Si3).

☞ For pain on the top of the head, add the following:
- ☞ Gently knead the point located at the center of the top of the head on the line connecting the two tips of your ears (Gv20).
- ☞ Gently press and knead the point located between the big toe and the second toe, two finger-widths up from the joint between the toes on the foot (Liv3).

Heartburn (Stomach Pain)

WHAT IS IT AND WHAT CAUSES IT?

Heartburn is also called gastro-esophageal reflux disease. The symptoms include a painful or burning sensation in the center of the chest, a feeling that food is coming back into the throat, or a sour or bitter taste in the mouth.

The main causes are bad eating habits, such as overeating, too much cold, raw food, and too much alcohol. It occurs when the gastric acid in your stomach backs up into the lower esophagus. The acid produces a burning sensation and discomfort. Another reason for the upper abdomen pain is from digestive tract diseases such as gastritis, stomach or duodenal (first part of the small intestine) ulcers, stomach spasms, gastroneurosis, and gastroptosis.

WHEN SHOULD YOU SEE A DOCTOR?

If you have frequent heartburn, see a doctor.

WHAT SHOULD YOU DO IN DAILY LIFE?

- Eat smaller amounts frequently.
- Wear loose clothes and belt. Don't allow anything restrictive or tight around your stomach.

WHAT SHOULDN'T YOU DO?

- Do not overeat anything. Do not eat two hours before your bedtime.
- Avoid alcohol, beer, coffee, orange juice, and tomato juice. Avoid soda when you have a meal.
- Avoid fatty or fried foods. Avoid spicy foods such as hot pepper, raw onion, and garlic.
- Do not lie down after a meal. Do not lie flat on the bed. Keep your body at a slightly upward-tilting angle. Don't exercise right after meals.
- Don't smoke.

Folk Remedies

- Chew some sesame seeds to stop the acid.
- Bake eggshells to dry. Grind into fine powder. Eat 1 tsp. with warm water before meals, twice a day. You can also use cuttlefish bone instead of eggshells.

- Bake dates until crunchy. Place three or four dates into a cup of boiled water. Wait until the water becomes red and drink three times a day after each meal.

Food Therapy

- Drink 1 cup of warm milk with 1 tsp. of ginger juice.
- Make a smoothie witha small apple and a raw potato. Take once daily.
- Eat 15 raw peanuts three times a day before meals.

Chinese Massage

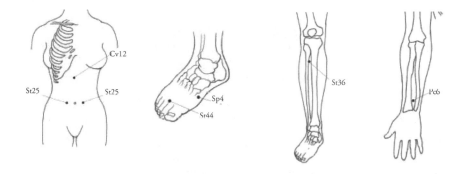

- Overlap your palms and rub around the belly button clockwise first, then counterclockwise 36 times respectively.
- Gently press and knead the following points for one minute:
  - The point halfway between your belly button and the lower edge of your breastbone (Cv12).
  - The point two thumb-widths above the wrist crease of the palm side, between the tendons, right under the buckle of the watchstrap (Pc6).

☞ The point two thumb-widths on either side of the belly button for one minute (St25).

☞ The depression four finger-widths below the kneecap edge and one thumb's-width outside of the shinbone (St36).

☞ The point on the inside of the foot in the depression behind the bone of the big toe (Sp4).

☞ The point on the base of toes between the second toe and the third toe (St44).

Chinese Herbs

☞ Take the patent herb Xiang Sha Yang Wei Wan. Follow the instructions.

Heel Pain (Chronic)

WHAT IS IT AND WHAT CAUSES IT?

The common cause of heel pain is an inflammation or small tear of the heel pad along the bottom of the foot. A pinched nerve or arthritis may cause heel pain also.

WHEN SHOULD YOU SEE A DOCTOR?

If your pain disrupts your daily life, or you feel no relief after self-treatment, see a doctor.

WHAT SHOULD YOU DO IN DAILY LIFE?

☞ Normal walking and jogging is fine. But walking or standing for a prolonged period is not good for heel pain.

☞ Wear soft shoes only. Do not wear high heels.

☞ Keep your feet warm in the winter.

WHAT SHOULDN'T YOU DO?

☞ Don't soak your heel in cold water.

Folk Remedies

- Place several golf or tennis balls in a shallow container and roll your bare feet over these balls for five minutes, three times a day.

- Soak your feet in water as hot as is comfortable for you and cold water alternately, each for five minutes.

- Use a big plastic soft drink bottle to gently knock your heel 50 times a day.

- Steam with rice vinegar:

    Ingredients: 500 ml vinegar, half a brick.

    Procedure: Place the brick in an oven or fireplace to warm it until it becomes hot. Soak the brick in the vinegar and place it about one foot beneath your feet. Steam your heel for five minutes. Be careful not to burn yourself.

- Use Chinese herb shoe pad:

    Ingredients: 1 oz. dang gui, 1/2 oz. ligusticum, 1/2 oz. mastic, 1/2 oz. gardenia.

    Procedure: Grind these herbs into a fine powder. Use cotton fabric to make two shoe pads. Place the herb powder in pads evenly. Use these two pads alternately. Place in shoes while wearing them.

Chinese Massage

- Using your palm knead, scrub, and press the heel, focus on the spot in pain for five minutes. Use the heel of your palm to gently knock that spot 10 times. Then gently knock the surrounding area 10 times.

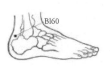

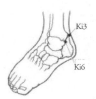

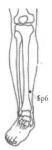

☞ Cross your legs by placing the ankle of the foot whose heel is bothersome on the other thigh. Using your fingers, knead, rub, and grasp from the back of the knee down to the heel, focusing on your heel tendon and the surrounding area for five minutes. Rotate your ankle clockwise and counterclockwise 10 times.

☞ Using your thumb, gently press the point located in the depression behind the top of the outside anklebone 10 times (Bl60).

☞ Using your thumb, gently press the depression behind the top of the inside anklebone 10 times (Ki3).

☞ Using your thumb, gently press and knead the point on the lower edge of the inside anklebone (Ki6).

☞ Using your thumb, gently press the point four finger-widths up from the inside anklebone, right behind the leg bone (Sp6).

Heat Therapy

☞ Light a smokeless moxa stick, available in Chinese herb stores. Circulate it 1 to 2 inches above the heel for five to 10 minutes. Do this two times a day. Take care not to burn yourself.

Chinese Herbs

☞ Take the patent herb Gu Zhi Zeng Sheng Wan. Follow the instructions.

Hemorrhoids

WHAT IS IT AND WHAT CAUSES IT?

Hemorrhoids are the swelling of the veins at the anal opening. The symptoms may include blood in the stool and the presence of painful lumps at the anus. Excess force during bowel movements and constipation are considered the main causes of hemorrhoids.

WHEN SHOULD YOU SEE A DOCTOR?

If you see bright blood in stool or on toilet paper, or there is no sign of improvement two weeks after self-treatment, see a doctor.

WHAT SHOULD YOU DO IN DAILY LIFE?

- Set a regular schedule for using the bathroom. The best time is 20 minutes after your breakfast. Use soft or premoistened toilet paper to clean yourself first. Then apply unscented moisturizing cream.
- Put ice in a plastic bag, wrap it with cloth, and sit on it for 10 minutes. It could help to reduce the acute inflammation.
- Take hot showers frequently.
- Eat a high-fiber diet, including foods such as celery, Chinese cabbage, yams, soybeans, or ripe bananas. Drink a lot of water every day.
- Exercise regularly. One reason for hemorrhoids is lack of exercise. Walking and jogging can make blood circulation better.
- If you have constipation or diarrhea, treat them promptly.

WHAT SHOULDN'T YOU DO?

- Avoid standing or sitting for long periods of time. Avoid walking with a heavy load for a prolonged time.
- Don't read a book when you are sitting on the toilet. Defecating too long will cause venous engorgement, which can lead to hemorrhoids.
- Do not strain or hold your breath on the toilet.
- Do not scratch the hemorrhoids.
- Avoid spicy and greasy food, hot peppers, garlic, onions, or pepper. Don't eat shrimp, crab, and lamb.
- If you have severe hemorrhoids, don't have sex too much. When you have sex, the muscles on the back and hip will constrict and press the vein around the anus constantly, blocking the blood circulation.

Folk Remedies

❧ Apply aloe vera: Mix aloe vera cream (84 percent) with aloe vera gel (98 percent). Apply to the anus when you have bleeding.

❧ Holding your body upside down can improve circulation of your vein blood in the pelvic cavity. Lying near a wall and using your shoulders, elbows, and head as support, raise your legs and buttocks up and stretch your body against the wall. Keep there for one or two minutes. Use belly breathing if you can. Do this three times a day. If you are elderly or you have any heart problems or any eye problems, don't use this method. Go to the bathroom before beginning this exercise. Don't do this if you are too hungry or too full.

❧ Jumping with single leg: Jump 20 times with one leg, then change to the other. This will increase circulation. Exercise for five to 10 minutes a day.

Food Therapy

❧ Eat tofu with sugar: Add half a slice of tofu and 1 Tbs. of sugar to a pot. Add enough water to just cover the tofu. Bring to a boil, reduce heat, and simmer for five minutes. Eat the tofu and the soup together in the morning on an empty stomach.

❧ Eat white and black fungus with dates: Soak 1/4 oz. of white fungus and 1/4 oz. of black fungus in water for three hours. Cook them with 10 red dates in a pot with 3 cups of water. Divide into two portions. Eat them twice a day for a week.

❧ Eat water chestnuts with brown sugar. Peel 2 oz. of chestnuts. Add 1 cup of water and 1/2 oz. of brown sugar. Bring to a boil. Reduce heat and simmer for three minutes. Eat once a day.

Chinese Massage

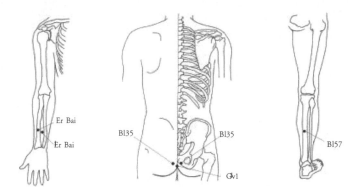

> ❧ Gently press and knead the point between the anus and the tip of the tailbone (Gv1). Press towards to the tailbone until your anus has a sensation of soreness and distention, then slowly release. Repeat for two minutes.

> ❧ Gently press and knead the point half a finger's-width from the tip of the tailbone on both sides for one minute (Bl35).

> ❧ Gently press and knead the point in the depression underneath the large muscle of the calf, about halfway between the knee crease and the heel for one minute (Bl57).

> ❧ Using your index and middle fingers gently press and knead the points on inside of the forearm four thumbwidths up from the crease of the wrist for one minute (Er Bai). There are two Er Bai for each arm.

Qi Gong

> ❧ Stand in a quiet room. Relax the whole body. Tuck the buttocks in. Concentrate your mind on the practice. Breathe naturally.

> ❧ When you inhale, place the thighs together with force and raise the tongue against the hard palate. At the same time, constrict and lift the anus as if to restrain defecation.

- ☞ Hold the breath for two seconds. Then exhale and relax the anus.
- ☞ Repeat this sequence for five minutes. Do this exercise two times a day.

Chinese Herbs

- ☞ Apply the patent herb called Ma Ying Long ointment. Follow the instructions.
- ☞ Take the patent herb called Di Yu Huai Jiao Wan. Follow the instructions.

High Blood Pressure (Hypertension)

WHAT IS IT AND WHAT CAUSES IT?

High blood pressure often has no symptoms. Nowadays, doctors recommend the ideal pressures to be below 120 for systolic and below 80 for diastolic. Your blood pressure fluctuates normally according to your activity. The arterioles play a very important role in regulating the blood pressure. If they are constricted, your blood pressure goes high. In most cases, the reason the regulatory system does not work well is unknown. Research shows stress, smoking, obesity, high intake of sodium, and genetic factors are related. High blood pressure can cause stroke, diabetes, coronary heart disease, and kidney disease.

WHEN SHOULD YOU SEE A DOCTOR?

Check blood pressure regularly. If you have a family history of hypertension or heart disease you need to check your blood pressure more frequently. If you do have hypertension, you should always be under a doctor's care for your lifestyle guidance or perhaps some medications.

WHAT SHOULD YOU DO IN DAILY LIFE?

- ☞ Take your medication faithfully and follow the prescription.
- ☞ Keep sodium intake low.
- ☞ Exercise daily. Research shows Tai Chi is an excellent choice in this situation. Walking in the rain is good too.

The negative ion calms you down and lowers your blood pressure. If your blood pressure is moderate, you can do aerobic exercise such as jogging or cycling. Walking up stairs is another choice.

- Eat your meals regularly. Eat more fresh vegetables and fruits, and eat more mushrooms, particularly Chinese dried mushroom or edible Chinese white and black fungus.

- Check your cholesterol regularly.

- Drink plenty of water. Green tea or mineral water is good for you. Drink only moderate amounts of red wine.

- Take a warm bath for 20 minutes every day. The key is the temperature, which should not be too high, about 100 degrees Fahrenheit. Remember to keep your bathroom warm, too. Walking out from warm bath water into a cold room will constrict your vessels.

- Wear warm and loose clothes. Cold makes your blood pressure higher. Your tie and belt should not be tight. Shoes should not be too heavy or too small. Wear a soft, warm hat in the wintertime.

- If you are elderly, you should speak less and listen more. Speaking loudly raises the blood pressure.

- If you are overweight, controlling your weight is crucial to lowering your blood pressure.

WHAT SHOULDN'T YOU DO?

- Don't be angry, which makes your blood pressure higher. Use distraction, talking out, restraint, or avoidance to get rid of your anger. Learn to use crying to relieve your grief and sadness.

- Don't see scary, thriller, or action movies, as any emotional fluctuation is not good for your blood pressure.

- Don't smoke.

- Avoid exposure to cold conditions.

- Don't miss your breakfast, or eat too much for dinner.

- Don't lower your blood pressure too quickly.

- Don't stop treatment when your blood pressure is back into the normal (healthy) range.

- Don't change your body position suddenly, particularly the elderly.
- Avoid constipation. Have regular bowel movements.

Folk Remedies

- Sleep on a chrysanthemum pillow:

    Ingredients: 20 oz. chrysanthemum flower, 8 oz. ligusticum, 4 oz. angelica, 4 oz. moutan bark, 4 oz. siler.

    Procedure: Use two layers of cotton fabric to make a bag. Fill with herbs. Change every six months. You can also use just chrysanthemum.

- Working on your feet:

    - Soak your feet in a foot spa. Add 1 oz. of baking soda into a tub with warm water. Soak your feet for 20 minutes, once a day. Add hot water to keep the temperature, being careful not to scald yourself. If you have an allergic reaction, discontinue use.

    - Sit on a chair. Place one leg over another. Rotate your ankle clockwise 20 times. Change legs and do the opposite side. Use your fingers to rotate each big toe 15 times. Massage your toes and then all over, focus on the point called "Blood Pressure Point." (See the illustration on page 162).

    - Use an empty, plastic soft drink bottle to gently knock both soles rhythmically for 10 minutes, especially focus on the point below the ball of the foot in the center, about a third of the distance between the toes and the heel (Ki1).

    - Place a vacuum cleaner pipe on the floor. Roll it back and forth with your soles and toes for 20 minutes.

- Do the following small trick whenever you have spare time:

    - Pinch all around the edge of the earlobe and the place behind the ear where it attaches to the head. Gently press the back of the ear.

☞ Rub and gently press your right palm from the center of the palm to the tip of the middle finger until you feel warm. Change hands and repeat this procedure.

Food Therapy

☞ Eat cooked bananas:

Ingredients: 1 ripe banana.

Procedure: Peel banana and cut into pieces. Place in a pan with 1 cup of water. Bring to boil. Simmer for 10 minutes. Eat one banana a day for a prolonged period.

☞ Eat peanuts soaked in vinegar:

Ingredients: 3 oz. peanuts with red skin, 300 ml rice vinegar.

Procedure: Soak the peanuts in vinegar for 15 days. Eat 10 pieces at a time, two times a day for a prolonged period. Be sure to brush teeth after eating.

☞ Drink lotus leaf soup:

Ingredients: 1/8 oz. dry lotus leaves (available in Chinese grocery stores).

Procedure: Clean the lotus leaves first. Soak them in water overnight. Cut them into pieces, add 2 cups of water and the leaves to a pot and bring to a boil. Reduce heat and simmer for 10 minutes. Divide into two portions for two days. Drink three times a day. Warm soup before drinking.

☞ Drink red small bean soup:

Ingredients: 2 oz. red small beans.

Procedure: Soak beans in 4 cups of water overnight. Put everything in a pot and bring to a boil. Reduce heat and simmer for one hour. Drink 100 ml (each time), three times a day.

☞ Drink salvia wine:

Ingredients: 4 oz. salvia, 1 bottle red wine.

Procedure: Soak the salvia in one bottle of red wine for 30 days. Drink 30 ml every morning and every evening.

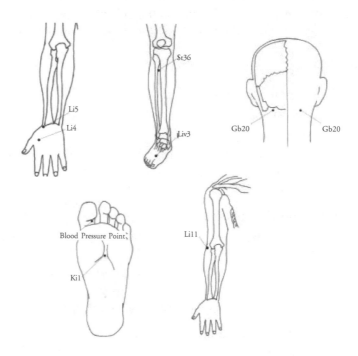

Chinese Massage

🖙 Bundle 10 toothpicks together to gently stimulate the following two points to lower blood pressure. Gently press for 10 minutes, twice a day:

   🖙 On the back of the hand in the depression, where the wrist crease meets the line from the thumb (Li5).

   🖙 With your thumb against the index finger, the webbing where it bulges up the highest (Li4).

🖙 Use the following techniques and massage once a day.

   🖙 Rub the forehead: Rub from the middle point between the two eyebrows, up to the front hairline of the forehead 30 times. Rub from the central line of the forehead to both sides 30 times.

- Knead the temple: Gently press the temple and circularly rub in a backwards direction 30 times. Press and knead the center point on the top of your head 30 times.
- Dry bathe the face: Rub your hands against each other until they are warm. Wipe with your palms from the top of the forehead, first sideways then downward, then rub in reverse, upward from the sides of the nose 30 times.
- Gently press and knead the point in the depression at the bottom of the skull, outside of the two big muscles on the neck, which you can feel by bending down your neck (Gb20).
- Gently press the point between the big and the second toe, two finger-widths up from the root of the toe, on the top of your foot (Liv3).
- Gently press the point at the end of the crease on the top of the elbow joint, when the arm is folded across the chest (Li11).
- Gently press the depression four finger-widths below the kneecap edge and one thumb's-width outside of the shinbone (St36).

Qi Gong

Do the following, step by step, and repeat three times. Take a rest after each cycle.

- Lie down. Slightly close your eyes. Take a deep breath.
- Tell yourself, "Both sides of my head are relaxed, both sides of my neck are relaxed, my shoulders are relaxed, my upper arms are relaxed, my forearms are relaxed, my wrists are relaxed, my hands are relaxed, my 10 fingers are relaxed."
- Tell yourself, "My face is relaxed, my neck is relaxed, my chest is relaxed, my abdomen is relaxed, my two thighs are relaxed, my knees are relaxed, my two feet are relaxed, my 10 toes are relaxed."
- Tell yourself, "The back of my head is relaxed, the back of my neck is relaxed, my back is relaxed, the back of my

waist is relaxed, the posterior parts of both thighs are relaxed, the backside of my knees are relaxed, my two calves are relaxed, the two soles of my feet are relaxed."

Chinese Herbs

☞ Drink dogbane tea:

Ingredients: 1/16 oz. dogbane.

Procedure: Add boiling water to make tea. Drink once a day.

☞ If you have blurred vision, dizziness, ear ringing, or insomnia, take the patent herb Zhi Bai Di Huang Wan. Follow the instructions.

☞ If you have a flushed face with red eyes, headache, or dry mouth with a bitter sensation, take the patent herb Niu Huang Jiang Ya Wan. Follow the instructions.

Hives (Urticaria)

WHAT IS IT AND WHAT CAUSES IT?

Hives are red, swollen wheals (welts) on the skin that are extremely itchy. Hives are an allergic reaction to many different factors such as tension, stress, food, medication, sunshine, or wind.

WHEN SHOULD YOU SEE A DOCTOR?

If you have hives, you need to see a doctor to determine what the real trigger is, particularly if you are taking medication for another illness. If you have hives in your throat and experience breathing and swallowing difficulties, see a doctor immediately.

WHAT SHOULD YOU DO IN DAILY LIFE?

☞ Keep a diary to find out the triggers and avoid them. The diary should include weather, clothing, food, activities, emotions, and so on.

* You can pat with your palm to soothe the itching. A cold bath or a cold compress may help relieve the itching, or try applying an ice cube for a few minutes for some relief from the itching.
* Watch your diet. Pay special attention to foods such as chicken, lamb, milk, seafood, tomatoes, onions, mushrooms, peanuts, beer, vinegar, chocolate, and fried food. If necessary, start your diet from a single food, gradually increasing items to find out which one is the trigger.

WHAT SHOULDN'T YOU DO?

* Don't scratch the infected spot. Don't use a hot bath or shower to wash the affected area.
* Don't wear clothing that is too tight or too warm. Don't wear wool or polyester clothes—these can irritate your skin.
* Don't eat spicy food or drink alcohol.

Folk Remedies

* Wash with salt water: Wash the affected area with warm water first. Dissolve 1 oz. of salt in 1 cup of boiled water. Wait until it cools a bit, then wash and rub the affected area repeatedly. Don't wash them off for three hours. (Do a skin test before trying this remedy.)
* Use a low-power vacuum cleaner to alleviate your itching: Remove the head or brush of the vacuum cleaner. Use the opening of the pipe to gently suck at your bellybutton (navel). Try to slightly lift the pipe, but don't lose contact with the skin. Continue for 10 seconds with suction. Repeat several times.

Food Therapy

* If the wheal is red and hot, take the following tea:
    Ingredients: 1 oz. peel of winter melon, 1/4 oz. chrysanthemum flower, 1/4 oz. red peony.

Procedure: Add 3 cups of water and ingredients to a pot and bring to a boil. Reduce heat and simmer for 15 minutes. Strain the decoction and add a bit of honey to drink as tea, once a day for five days.

☞ If the wheal is white, take the following tea:

Ingredients: 1/4 oz. ginger, 1 oz. crystal sugar.

Procedure: Place the ginger in a pot with 2 cups of water. Bring to a boil. Reduce heat and simmer for 10 minutes. Add sugar and drink one batch two times a day for five days.

☞ If your symptoms become worse with over exertion or the attacks repeat over and over with dry mouth and irritability, take the following tea:

Ingredients: 1/4 oz. black sesame seeds, 1/2 oz. black dates, 1 oz. black beans.

Procedure: Soak beans in water overnight. Place all ingredients in a pot with 2 cups of water. Bring to a boil. Reduce heat and simmer until beans are soft. Eat them all, once a day, for five days.

Chinese Massage

Massage the following points on both sides once a day:

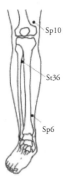
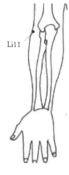

- ✒ Use the thumb to gently press the point at the end of the crease on the top of the elbow joint, when the arm is folded across the chest for one minute (Li11).
- ✒ Use the middle finger to gently press the depression four finger-widths below the kneecap edge and one thumb's-width outside of the shinbone for one minute (St36).
- ✒ Gently press and knead the point four finger-widths up from the inside anklebone, right behind the leg bone for one minute (Sp6).
- ✒ Gently press the point on the top of the inside edge of the knee for one minute. (Flex your knee and place your hand on the kneecap. The point is where your thumb touches (Sp10).

Chinese Herbs

- ✒ Eat chicken with herb:

    Ingredients: 3 oz. chicken without bone, 1/16 oz. pseudoginseng, 1 tsp. cooking oil.

    Procedure: Slice pseudoginseng and stir-fry with cooking oil until it becomes yellowish. Slice chicken meat and mix with the herb. Place in a bowl and steam for one hour. Add a bit of salt and eat it once a day for three days.

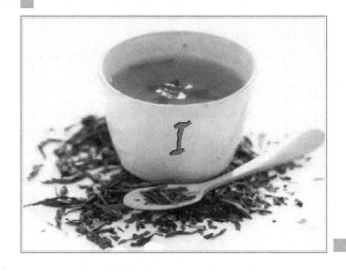

Impotence

WHAT IS IT AND WHAT CAUSES IT?

Impotence is the inability to achieve and maintain an erection during sexual intercourse. Many physical and psychological factors can cause the problem such as artery problems, nerve disorders, heart disease, diabetes, anxiety, depression, and the side effects of medications.

WHEN SHOULD YOU SEE A DOCTOR?

If you persistently have difficulty in achieving or maintaining an erection, or if you found this problem after taking a medication, see a doctor.

WHAT SHOULD YOU DO IN DAILY LIFE?

- Reduce stress and relax. Anxiety about performing is the main cause of impotence.
- Eat more lamb, walnuts, black beans, bone soup, dates, sesame seeds, and lotus seeds, which, according to

Chinese medicine, will strengthen male potency. Eat zinc-rich foods such as oysters, beef, and eggs. Eat more arginine-rich food such as Chinese yams, frozen tofu, squid, and cuttlefish.

* If you have a prostate problem, treat it promptly.

WHAT SHOULDN'T YOU DO?

* Don't have sex too much if you feel weak physically. Too much sex is another common factor of impotence. During the treatments for your impotence, don't have sex.
* Don't drink alcohol. Alcoholics have higher than normal rate of erectile disorders.
* Stop smoking. Long-term smoking will reduce the blood circulation in the penis.
* Don't wear tight pants or ride a bicycle too long. Pressure or friction on the genitals will not help impotence.
* Don't overexert and get enough sleep.
* Reduce cholesterol intake.
* Don't be shy about seeing a doctor for your problem. A wife or significant other should encourage a partner to do so.

Folk Remedy

* Apply ginger and fennel fruit on the belly button:
  Ingredients: 1/4 oz. fennel fruits, 1/4 oz. ginger, honey.
  Procedure: Stir fry ginger on low heat until dark. Grind fennel fruits and ginger into fine powders. Mix ginger and fruits with a little bit of honey to make a paste. Apply to your belly button and seal with a bandage. Keep for three hours a day for a week. If you have an allergic reaction, discontinue use immediately.

Food Therapy

* Eat walnuts and chestnuts: Crush 1/2 oz. of each of them and add 1 tsp. of sugar. Eat once a day.

☙ Take prawn wine:

> **Ingredients:** 12 oz. prawn, 180 ml 80-proof vodka, 360 ml Chinese cooking wine.
>
> **Procedure:** Wash the prawns first. Soak them in a sealed bottle with vodka for one day. Discard the vodka. Use cooking wine to cook the prawns for two minutes (most of the alcohol will burn off). Divide into two portions. Eat the prawns and drink the cooking wine once a day for two days. Repeat three times.

☙ Drink seahorse wine:

> **Ingredients:** A pair of seahorses (available in Chinese herb stores), 500 ml 80-proof vodka.
>
> **Procedure:** Wash seahorse and dry them. Soak them sealed in vodka for two weeks. Mix 15 ml water with 15 ml herbal vodka. Drink before bedtime.

☙ Drink herb wine:

> **Ingredients:** 4 oz. epimedium, 500 ml 80-proof vodka.
>
> **Procedure:** Crush the epimedium and put it into a sterilized cotton fabric bag. Soak it in vodka. Seal the container for three days. Mix 15 ml water with 15 ml herbal vodka. Drink it two times a day.

☙ Eat river shrimp stir-fried with Chinese chives:

> **Ingredients:** 4 oz. Chinese chives, 8 oz. river shrimp, 1 Tbs. cooking oil, salt.
>
> **Procedure:** Cut chives into 1-inch long pieces. Stir-fry the chives and the river shrimp in cooking oil with 1/2 tsp. of salt. Eat twice a week.

☙ Eat lamb with garlic:

> **Ingredients:** 8 oz. lamb, 1/2 oz. garlic.
>
> **Procedure:** Cook lamb with 2 cups of water until it is well done, then slice and mix with the crushed garlic. Add some soy sauce and cayenne to eat.

Chinese Massage

Choose the following and massage once a day.

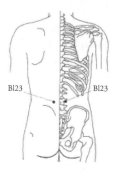 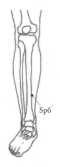 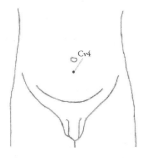

☞ Sit on a chair. Place both hands on the midline of your back. Scrub down to the tailbone 100 times until you feel a warm sensation. Use both palms to rub and push the low back and sacral bone.

☞ Use your fingers to gently press the points a little higher than the waist, two finger-widths on both sides of the spine for two minutes (Bl23).

☞ Use your thumb to gently press and knead the point on the midline of the abdomen, four finger-widths below the belly button (navel) for one minute (Cv4). Use your fingers to gently press the dent right above the root of the penis for one minute.

☞ Place your right palm on the root of the testicles. Lift testicles and penis up a bit. Use your left palm to gently press the area right bellow the belly button. Meanwhile constrict the sphincter muscles of the anus. Repeat 20 times.

☞ Lie down on your back. Use both palms to push from the breastbone down toward the pubic bone 100 times. Start very gently, and gradually increase the pressure.

☞ Use your fingers to gently press and knead the point four finger-widths up from the inside anklebone, right behind the leg bone for one minute (Sp6).

Chinese Herbs

- If your impotence is caused by stress or other emotional factors, take the patent herb Xiao Yao Wan. Follow the instructions.
- If you have a pale complexion, soreness of back, or a cold sensation in the penis, abdomen, and limbs, take the patent herb Nan Bao. Follow the instructions.
- If your erectile function is normal in daily life, but fails before entering the vagina/intercourse, take the patent herb Zhi Bai Di Huang Wan. Follow the instructions.

Infertility for Females

WHAT IS IT AND WHAT CAUSES IT?

Infertility is defined as an inability to get pregnant after a full year of trying to conceive. Some possible causes include problems with ovulation, hormonal imbalance, endometriosis, and abnormalities in the reproductive organs.

WHEN SHOULD YOU SEE A DOCTOR?

If after one year's effort you are not pregnant, you and your spouse both should see a doctor.

WHAT SHOULD YOU DO IN DAILY LIFE?

- Eat nutritiously so that your uterine lining is healthy and capable of implanting a fertilized egg.
- Participate in non-intensive exercise such as Tai Chi and walking.
- Reduce both physical and mental stress. They could interfere with the pregnancy process.
- Seize the window of opportunity for pregnancy. Use an ovulation test kit to determine the time of your ovulation. Have sex during the time starting two to three days before and 24 hours after the time of ovulation.

WHAT SHOULDN'T YOU DO?

- ❧ Don't be overanxious. This goes for the man as well as the woman. Anxiousness can interfere with the production and secretion of sperm and the function of the fallopian tubes. This is the reason why after giving up trying and adopting a baby, some couples then conceive unexpectedly.

- ❧ Don't have frequent sex, especially before the time that holds the best chance for conception. Man needs time for his sperm count to rise back to normal after sex.

- ❧ Don't drink alcohol, smoke, or eat too much overstimulatory food such as hot peppercorn, garlic, or ginger.

Folk Remedies

- ❦ Puncture a small hole in an egg and put in 1/16 oz. of saffron (available in Chinese herb stores). Shake the egg to thoroughly mix the content, then steam the egg to well done. Eat one egg a day for the nine days after your period arrives.

- ❦ Get donkey-hide gelatin and grind it into a fine powder. Eat 1/8 oz. at a time together with 50 ml rice wine a day.

Heat Therapy

- ❦ Use a lighted smokeless moxa stick, which is like a cigar and is available in Chinese herb stores, to smoke the following points. Do so two times a day, 15 minutes each time. Be careful not to burn yourself.
  - ☙ On the midline of the abdomen four finger-widths below the belly button (Cv4).
  - ☙ On the middle of the abdomen two finger-widths below the belly button (Cv6).
  - ☙ The point four finger-widths up from the inside anklebone, right behind the leg bone (Sp6).
  - ☙ The depression four finger-widths below the kneecap edge and one thumb's-width outside of the shinbone (St36).

Chinese Massage

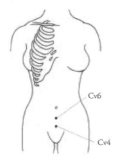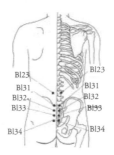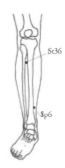

- ☞ Place your right palm below the belly button. Gently rub clockwise for one minute. Gradually increase the pressure.
- ☞ Place the pad of the thumb on the points a little higher than the waist, two finger-widths on both sides of the spine (Bl23). Gently press the area for two minutes.
- ☞ Use the tips of your index, middle, ring, and little fingers to tap the sacrum area, right along the central line (Bl31-Bl34) for one minute.
- ☞ Place both of your palms on the sacrum area. Scrub from bottom up until you have a warm sensation.
- ☞ Use your thumb or index finger to gently press and knead these points mentioned in previous "heat therapy" section for one minute.

Chinese Herbs

- ☞ If you have small, dark but clear-of-clots menstrual flow, prolonged periods, or coldness in the low abdomen, take the patent herb You Gui Wan. Follow the instructions.
- ☞ If you have irregular periods with fluctuated menstrual flow, bloating sensations in the breasts, melancholy, or irritability, take the patent herb Xiao Yao Wan. Follow the instructions.

☞ If you have delayed periods with small and light-color menstrual flow, a pale complexion, or weight loss, take the patent herb Wu Ji Bai Feng Wan. Follow the instructions.

☞ If you are obese, have irregular periods, and feel fullness in the chest, take the patent herb Er Chen Wan. Follow the instructions.

☞ If you have serious pain during your period worsened by applying pressure, and dark and purplish clots in menstrual flow, take the patent herb Dang Gui Wan. Follow the instructions.

Infertility for Males

WHAT IS IT AND WHAT CAUSES IT?

It is the inability to achieve pregnancy after one year of trying to conceive. The main cause of male infertility is impaired sperm production. Chronic anxiety can have a major impact on conception.

WHEN SHOULD YOU SEE A DOCTOR?

If after one year your wife or significant other doesn't become pregnant, you both should see a doctor.

WHAT SHOULD YOU DO IN DAILY LIFE?

❧ You should try to have a relaxed and optimistic outlook and don't become overstressed.

❧ Proper nutrition also plays a role.

❧ Consult with your doctor to see if any medication has affected your sperm levels.

WHAT SHOULDN'T YOU DO?

❧ Don't smoke. If you smoke, your sperm density and mobility is much lower than normal.

- Eat less celery. Research shows too much celery will decrease the quantity of the sperm.
- Don't take hot baths frequently and don't wear underwear that is too tight. Don't ride a bicycle too long. Try to keep your testicles at a lower temperature because excessive heat in this area can be adverse to sperm formation.
- Don't work with a laptop on your thighs for long periods of time because it can raise the temperature of testicles.

Food Therapy

- Eat lamb with herbs:

   Ingredients: 3 oz. lamb, 1/8 oz. epimedium, 1/8 oz. Siberian olomonseal rhizome.

   Procedure: Wrap herbs in gauze. Slice lamb into small chunks. Add 2 cups of water and cook until lamb is soft. Add seasoning and eat the lamb once a day.

- Drink walnuts and rice soup:

   Ingredients: 3 oz. walnuts, 4 oz. rice, 1 oz. lycium fruit.

   Procedure: Crush walnuts into small pieces. Add walnuts and rice to 3 cups of water, bring to a boil and reduce heat to simmer for 20 minutes. At the last minute add the lycium fruit. Eat once a day.

Chinese Massage

Choose the following and massage once a day:

- Sit on a chair. Place both hands on the midline of your back. Scrub down to the tailbone until you have a warm sensation.
- Use your fingers to gently press the points a little higher to the waist, two finger-widths on both sides of the spine for two minutes (Bl23).

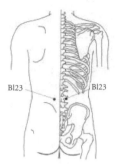 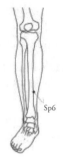 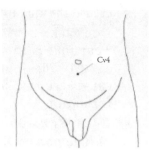

☞ Use your thumb to gently press and knead the point on the midline of the abdomen, four finger-widths below the belly button for one minute (Cv4).

☞ Use your fingers to gently press and knead the point four finger-widths up from the inside anklebone, right behind the leg bone for one minute (Sp6).

Chinese Herbs

☞ If you have dizziness, irritability, thick semen, ear ringing, warm sensations in the palm and soles, weak back and knees, or memory problems, take the patent herb Liu Wei Di Huang Wan. Follow the instructions.

☞ If you have lower sexual drive, impotence, and aversion to cold, take the patent herb Jin Gui Shen Qi Wan. Follow the instructions.

☞ If you have a low sex drive, thin semen, both physical and mental exhaustion, and a pale complexion, take the patent herb Shi Quan Da Bu Wan. Follow the instructions.

☞ If you have impotence, thick and yellowish semen possibly with blood, and a bloated abdomen, take the patent herb Er Miao Wan. Follow the instructions.

☞ If you have sensations of soreness and bloating in the abdomen, drooping and painful testicles, thick semen, and depression, take the patent herb Ju He Wan. Follow the instructions.

Insomnia

WHAT IS IT AND WHAT CAUSES IT?

Insomnia is the inability to fall asleep or get enough sleep. It is a symptom caused by many psychological and medical disorders such as depression, kidney failure, heart disease, and asthma. Your age and the medication you take also play a role in insomnia.

WHEN SHOULD YOU SEE A DOCTOR?

If constant insomnia is affecting your daily life, or your self-treatment is not working, see a doctor.

WHAT SHOULD YOU DO IN DAILY LIFE?

- Set a definite time to go to sleep and awaken. Don't violate the schedule even on weekends and holidays. Your body's circadian rhythm needs to be regular.
- Soak your feet up to the calves for 15 minutes in warm water one hour before bedtime daily. The temperature is between 104 degrees Fahrenheit and 110 degrees Fahrenheit.
- Combing your scalp frequently, which is equal to massage, can help.
- Eat more zinc-rich and copper-rich foods such as fish, oyster, lean meat, peanuts, dairy products, crab, lamb, peas, broad beans, and mushrooms. Lack of these minerals may cause insomnia for women.
- Practice Tai Chi or walk slowly for 30 minutes two hours before bedtime. Both are good exercises to overcome insomnia.
- Control your room temperature at 60 degress Fahrenheit. If the temperature is over 75 degrees Fahrenheit you are more likely to wake up at night. Use a heavy curtain to block light from other sources.
- Have sex to reduce tension. Sex also releases endorphins to help you sleep.

WHAT SHOULDN'T YOU DO?

- ⋇ Don't eat a heavy meal in the evening, especially right before bedtime. The interval between the meal and sleep should be four hours.

- ⋇ Don't worry if you can't go to sleep. Don't repeatedly look at the clock if you can't fall asleep. Turn the clock's face away from you and don't use a clock that has a too-bright LCD display.

- ⋇ Don't take sleeping pills after drinking alcohol.

- ⋇ Don't drink alcohol, coffee, or strong tea in the evening.

- ⋇ Don't smoke before bedtime.

- ⋇ Don't read books or perform tasks that are taxing on the brain before bedtime.

Folk Remedies

- ☙ Place an open bag with fresh orange peel, banana peel, or finely sliced ginger beside your pillow. Or place a little bag of lavender or jasmine beside your pillow. The aroma coming from these substances have soothing effects.

- ☙ When you are in bed, try one of the following:

  - ⋇ Lie down on your back. Place both hands together just like the Buddha's prayer. Rub them together until they are warm. Go back to a normal position. Slightly raise both of your knees and place both of your feet together, sole against sole. Rub your soles against each other until they are warm. Go back to a normal position. Repeat above exercises five times, and you may begin to feel drowsy.

  - ⋇ Close your eyes. Place hands beside you. Bend your fingers to slowly make a fist, then slowly open it. The frequency is about 30 seconds for one cycle. Keep your mind on the movement. Slow down the pace gradually until you fall asleep.

☞ Treating your feet or legs can balance your autonomic system and help you sleep:

   ☞ Gently tap your soles and both sides of the feet with a hairbrush for five minutes. The hairbrush acts like a bunch of acupuncture needles to stimulate the meridian and prompt the circulation of Qi and blood. Pay special attention to the point below the ball of the foot in the center, about a third of the distance between the toes and the heel.

   ☞ Before bedtime, heat a big bowl of soybeans in a microwave until hot but comfortable to the touch. Put the beans in a shallow container. Roll your feet in the container and massage your feet with these beans.

   ☞ When you are watching TV, use a big, plastic soft drink bottle to gently tap the depression four finger-widths below the kneecap edge and one thumb's-width outside the shinbone (St36). (See page 182.)

☞ Play the Chinese health balls with your hands for 20 minutes. The balls are available at Chinese herb stores. You can use one ball at a time for 10 to 15 minutes, or simultaneously with two balls. Do this several times a day for a prolonged period of time. This kind of exercise has many benefits and is good for the elderly.

Food Therapy

☞ Drink a cup of warm milk, or soymilk with honey, one hour before bedtime.

☞ Drink a small bowl of millet soup with 1 tsp. of sugar every night.

☞ Drink a cup of cold water with 1 tsp. of rice vinegar one hour before bedtime. If you have stomach problems, do not drink.

☞ Drink lucid ganoderma vodka:

   Ingredients: 1 oz. lucid ganoderma, 500 ml 80-proof vodka.

Procedure: Soak ganoderma in vodka in a sealed bottle for a week. Mix 20 ml water with 20 ml herbal vodka and drink at dinnertime.

☞ Eat lycium fruit with honey:

Ingredients: lycium fruit, honey.

Procedure: Soak lycium fruit in honey for 10 days. Eat 15 pieces of lycium fruit with 1 tsp. of honey three times a day for a month.

Chinese Massage

Massage the following once a day:

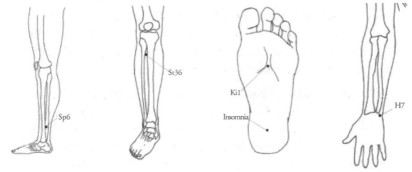

☞ Open your fingers and gently comb from the midline on the top of your head down to both cheeks for two minutes. Use the tips of your fingers together to gently tap the top of your head for two minutes. From the top center of the head slowly move to left, to right, to front, and to back. The key word is "gently."

☞ Gently press and knead the depression at the meeting point of the wrist crease of the palm side and the line from the little finger for one minute (H7). Change hands and do the other side.

☞ Gently press and knead the point four finger-widths up from the inside anklebone, right behind the leg bone for one minute (Sp6).

☞ Gently press and knead the point below the ball of the foot in the center, about a third of the distance between the toes and the heel for one minute (Ki1).

Qi Gong

Do "river of harmonious spirit" exercise. See **Anxiety** section.

Chinese Herbs

☞ Take 1/6 oz. of zizyphus granules with 1 cup of warm water, twice a day at around 5 p.m. and before bedtime.

Irritable Bowel Syndrome

WHAT IS IT AND WHAT CAUSES IT?

Irritable bowel syndrome is a collection of symptoms that range from bloating, diarrhea, and constipation to abdominal pain, all caused by the irritation of the large intestine. The precise cause of irritable bowel syndrome is not known, but it is often linked to stress, anxiety, or depression.

WHEN SHOULD YOU SEE A DOCTOR?

When you are chronically experiencing the previously mentioned symptoms, see a doctor.

WHAT SHOULD YOU DO IN DAILY LIFE?

☞ When taking showers in the morning, blast water at the abdomen. This kind of hot water massage will improve circulation and digestion.

☞ To combat stress, you can follow several methods. Practicing Qi Gong or Tai Chi can reduce stress. Pay attention to activities that seem to trigger the symptoms and try to avoid them.

☞ Sleep is the key. If you have an adequate amount of sleep, you can relieve some of the stress.

WHAT SHOULDN'T YOU DO?

- Don't drink coffee or alcohol because they will stimulate the already sensitive lining of the intestines.
- Don't eat spicy or fried food because they are difficult to digest and will add to the burden of the digestive system.
- Don't eat too much cold food. Extra energy will be needed to warm up the food as it is digested, which adds to the burden of the system.

Folk Remedies

- Every night, two hours before bedtime, place a hot wet towel on your stomach, followed by a layer of clear plastic wrap, and then a heating pad. Leave on for 20 minutes.

Food Therapy

- Eat a serving of yogurt every day. This helps maintain a healthy population of bacteria necessary for the digestive system.
- Egg with vinegar:

    Ingredients: 1 egg, 1/2 oz. ginger, 15 ml rice vinegar.

    Procedure: Put the ginger in a juicer with vinegar to make juice. Beat the egg. Mix egg with ginger juice. Stir well and cook for five seconds. Slowly sip the mixture once a day for three days.

Chinese Massage

- Use your palm to rub and knead your abdomen in a counterclockwise direction for three minutes. Start at the belly button and gradually move outward.
- Place both palms on your back. Rub down to the sacrum until you have a warm sensation in the abdomen.

🖎 Gently press the following points for one minute:

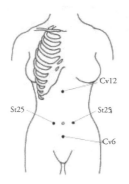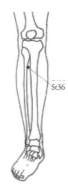

  🖎 The point halfway between the belly button and the lower edge of the breastbone (Cv12).

  🖎 The point on two finger-widths below the belly button on the midline of the abdomen (Cv6).

  🖎 The point two thumb-widths from your belly button (navel) on either side (St25).

  🖎 The depression four finger-widths below the kneecap edge and one thumb's-width outside of the shinbone (St36).

Chinese Herbs

🖎 If you have bloating and pain in the stomach that radiates to both ribs, belching, reflux, and a poor appetite, take the patent herb Si Ni San and Chai Hu Shu Gan Wan. Follow the instructions.

🖎 If you have a continuous, dull pain in the belly, that is worse with an empty stomach, and better with warmth, belching, or vomiting, take the patent herb Xiang Sha Liu Jun Zi Wan. Follow the instructions.

🖎 If you have stomach pain with a warm sensation, that is worse with eating, thirst, and irritability, take the patent herb Yi Guan Jian or Zuo Jin Wan. Follow the instructions.

Itching Dry Skin (Winter Itch)

WHAT IS IT AND WHAT CAUSES IT?

It is dry, itching skin with scaling, flaking, chapping, and irritation. This is usually caused (in the elderly especially) by winter weather.

WHEN SHOULD YOU SEE A DOCTOR?

If the itching bothers you persistently or you have a rash, see a doctor.

WHAT SHOULD YOU DO IN DAILY LIFE?

- Take enough vitamins.
- Wear cotton clothes. Wool or synthetic fabric next to the skin will cause itching.
- Use a mild soap, or liquid soap.
- Moisturize your body after a bath or shower with greasy moisturizers.
- Moisturize your room with a humidifier.
- Drink at least 8 cups of water a day. Eat more salmon, walnuts, and avocado. Drink less coffee, soda, and black tea.

WHAT SHOULDN'T YOU DO?

- Don't scratch. Instead, use a towel soaked in cold milk to apply to the affected area.
- Don't stand by a fireplace too long.
- Bathe no more than 15 minutes at a time, no more than three times a week. Use warm water instead of hot. Add 1 cup of cornstarch or ground fine oatmeal to bath water.
- Don't eat seafood or spicy food.
- No drinking alcohol or smoking.

Folk Remedies

🌿 Rub your affected area with banana peels or watermelon peels. Also add banana peels to water and cook, then use a towel soaked with banana water to wash the affected area.

🌿 Apply sliced apple on the itchy skin several times a day.

🌿 Rub with aloe vera: Cut the needles first. Slice it into two pieces from the center. Use the juicy side to rub the itching spot. If you have an allergic reaction, discontinue use.

Food Therapy

🌿 Drink kelp and mung bean soup:

Ingredients: 1/2 oz. kelp (dried seaweed), 2 oz. mung beans, sugar.

Procedure: Soak mung beans and kelp in water overnight. Place them in a pot with 3 cups of water and bring to a boil. Reduce heat and simmer until the beans become very soft. Add sugar, eat the kelp and beans, and drink the soup once a day for five days.

🌿 Drink edible white fungus soup:

Ingredients: 1 oz. Chinese white fungus, 2 oz. sugar.

Procedure: Soak the fungus in a bowl of water until it becomes very puffy. Wash the fungus very carefully. Place the fungus in a pot with 3 cups of water. Bring to a boil. Reduce heat and simmer for 10 minutes. Add sugar and divide into two portions. Eat twice a day for three days.

Chinese Herbs

🌿 Drink green tea with herbs:

Ingredients: 1/4 oz. licorice, 1/8 oz. talc, 1 tsp. green tea leaves.

Procedure: Place herbs in a pot, add 2 cups of water, and bring to a boil. Reduce heat and simmer for 20 minutes. Use the decoction to brew the green tea leaves. Drink a batch each day for three days.

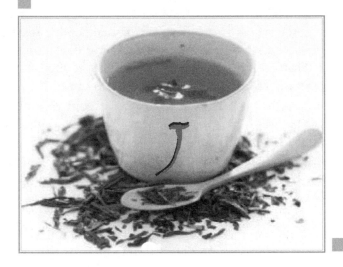

Jet Lag

WHAT IS IT AND WHAT CAUSES IT?

Tired yet unable to sleep; hungry yet unable to eat. Our bodies have a built-in biological clock to regulate the sleep/wakefulness cycle. It has trouble adjusting to the rapid time zone shifts made possible by air travel. The resulting fatigue and insomnia can sometimes take days or weeks to dissipate.

WHAT SHOULD YOU DO IN DAILY LIFE?

* Plan ahead to adjust to the change in time zones. Four days before the start of the trip, adjust your schedule to fit to the new time zone.

* Practice so-called "light therapy," which is spending some specific time in the sun to adjust your biological clock. If you fly from Los Angeles to London, four days before you leave do more outdoor activities from 9 a.m. to 2 p.m. It will gradually move your biological clock forward and change your bedtime from 10 p.m. to 8 p.m. If you

189

fly from New York to Hong Kong, do more outdoor activities after 2 p.m. Change your wakeup time from 6 a.m. to 8 a.m.

*   You can ease your transition by drinking coffee or tea at the time corresponding to the morning of the destination. Drink 1 cup of soymilk with honey at the time corresponding to the bedtime of the destination.

*   Strictly follow the regular schedule at your destination: Go to bed on time. Use some sleeping herbs if necessary (refer to **Insomnia** section). When you are awake in the middle of the night due to jet lag, you need to remain lying. If you are bored, listen to relaxing music or the radio. By resting according to the schedule of the new time zone, you can make the transition easier.

*   When you are feeling sleepy from jet lag, and it's still not close to bedtime, start doing things that are guaranteed to keep you awake. This can be socializing, exercises, or other activities you enjoy.

WHAT SHOULDN'T YOU DO?

*   Don't eat spicy food in an airplane at night.
*   Don't drink alcohol.

Folk Remedies

*   At your destination, when you sleep, put some dried chrysanthemum on your pillow. The herb helps to tranquilize you.

*   At your destination, apply a few drops of jasmine oil on your temples to help you go to sleep.

Chinese Massage

See **Insomnia** section.

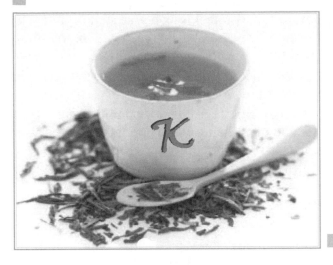

Knee Pain (Chronic)

WHAT IS IT AND WHAT CAUSES IT?

The knee joint and kneecap are swollen and stiff with the inability to move. Along with aging, knee pain can be caused by injury, sprain and strains, torn cartilage, osteoarthritis, runner's knee, tendonitis, or bursitis.

WHEN SHOULD YOU SEE A DOCTOR?

If you have pain or swelling in the knee, or you hear a buckling sound when you injure the knee, see a doctor.

WHAT SHOULD YOU DO IN DAILY LIFE?

- If it is caused by an injury, apply ice for 15 to 20 minutes first. Loosely wrap an elastic bandage to compress the area and raise your limb for 20 minutes. Repeat this procedure three to four times a day until the swelling disappears. After that, use a heating pad.

- In chronic cases, take a hot bath with Epsom salts. Follow the instructions. Add 2 oz. of 100-proof vodka if you want to. Gradually add hot water into the tub to a temperature that you feel is as hot as comfortable. Don't let the water level rise above your heart. If you are elderly or you have a heart condition, don't do this exercise.
- Keep the knee warm. Cut a piece of soft wool material and sew it into your pants.
- In osteoarthritis cases , take vitamin D, fish oil, and glucosamine chondroitin for a prolonged period to rebuild the cartilage and tendons.
- Control your weight to reduce the burden on the knee.

WHAT SHOULDN'T YOU DO?

- If you have knee problems, don't hike, climb, cycle, or do other intense physical activities, which put high stress on your knees. Instead, try swimming.
- Don't kneel or do full squats. Use a cane or other object to support your body when you try to stand up.

Folk Remedies

- Rub with liquor mixed with chili pepper:

  Ingredients: 200 ml 80-proof vodka, 2 oz. dehydrated small chili pepper.

  Procedure: Soak the pepper in the vodka for one week. Apply to the painful spot twice a day. If you have an allergic reaction, discontinue use.

- Apply hot salt: Use cotton fabric to make a book-size bag. Fill with cotton about 1-inch thick. Stir-fry 2 lbs. of salt for five minutes on low heat. Put the salt into the bag and seal it. Place the bag on the painful spot and cover with a blanket for one hour. Continue for one week. Take care not to burn yourself.

- Take a charcoal bath:

  Ingredients: 8 oz. charcoal (available in garden supply or barbeque supply stores).

Procedure: Boil the charcoal in hot water for 10 minutes. Take them out and wait for them to dry. Place them in a cotton fabric bag and put the bag in your bathtub. Soak your knee in warm water for 30 minutes. Do it once a day for one month. You can dry the charcoal for reuse.

☞ Gently tap your feet and leg with a hairbrush for five to 10 minutes after a warm bath. The hairbrush acts like a bunch of acupuncture needles to stimulate the meridian and prompt the circulation of Qi and blood.

    ☞ Tap the soles and both sides of your feet, from the heel to the toes. Pay more attention to the point below the ball of the foot in the center, about 1/3 of the distance between the toes and the heel (Ki1). (See page 194.)

    ☞ Tap each toe.

    ☞ Tap the back of your leg, from the lower part of your calf, up to the back of your thigh.

    ☞ Tap the area around your knee.

☞ Wash with vinegar and green onion:

Ingredients: 300 ml rice vinegar, 300 ml water, 1 lb. green onion.

Procedure: Cut green onion into 1-inch long pieces. Place in a pot with vinegar and water and bring to a boil. Use a piece of gauze dipped in this liquid to gently wash your knee for 10 minutes, two times a day. If the vinegar becomes cool, reheat it. If you have an allergic reaction, discontinue use.

Food Therapy

☞ Eat pearl barley soup:

Ingredients: 2 oz. Chinese pearl barley, 1 Tbs. sugar.

Procedure: Soak the barley in water overnight. Add barley and 2 cups of water to a pot and bring to a boil. Cook on low heat until the barley is soft. Add sugar. Eat once a day for two weeks.

☞ Eat chicken wing soup:

Ingredients: 1 lb. chicken wings, 3 slices ginger, 1/4 oz. onion, 1 lemon, salt, pepper.

Procedure: In a pot, add enough water to cover all wings and bring to a boil. Reduce heat and simmer approximately two hours. Remove the oil on the surface. Add salt, pepper, ginger, and lemon. Divide into three portions. Eat one portion at a time once a day.

Chinese Massage

In an acute case, don't massage your painful spot.

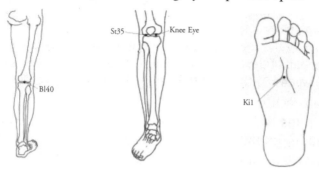

- Using your palm, rub and knead your kneecap for one minute.
- Using your palms, rub-roll both sides of your knee from the thigh down to your calf for one minute.
- Using your thumb, gently press and knead the painful spot for two minutes.
- Using your index finger, gently press and knead the point in the middle of the crease on the back of the knee when the knee is slightly bent (Bl40). Do this for one minute.
- Using your thumb, press into the two dents at the bottom of the kneecap, one on each side of the center. Do this for one minute (St35, Knee Eye).
- Using your thumb and fingers, grasp and knead the muscles on the front of your thigh and on the back of your lower leg for two minutes.

Chinese Herbs

- Take the patent herb Du Huo Ji Sheng Wan. Follow the instructions.
- Apply the herb patch Shang Shi Zhi Tong Gao to the painful spot. If you have an allergic reaction, discontinue use.

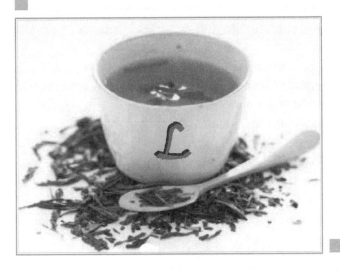

Laryngitis

WHAT IS IT AND WHAT CAUSES IT?

When the larynx is inflamed it is laryngitis. Its symptoms are sore throat, hoarseness, and difficulty making sounds. Laryngitis can be caused by many factors such as a viral infection or overuse of your voice, smoking, sinusitis, bronchitis, or exposure to some kind of chemical, dust, or other irritants.

WHEN SHOULD YOU SEE A DOCTOR?

If you have hoarseness and sore throat lasting more than two days, see a doctor. If the symptoms are accompanied with coughing up blood, painful swallowing, shortness of breath, or high fever, see a doctor immediately.

WHAT SHOULD YOU DO IN DAILY LIFE?

- Resting your voice is most important. Even whispering can make laryngitis worse.
- Drink eight to 10 glasses of water a day to lubricate the vocal cords.

195

* Use a facial steamer (available in a healthcare section of department stores) to lubricate your throat for 10 minutes, twice a day. Take care not to scald yourself.

* Use a cold-air humidifier to keep adequate humidity in your room.

* Apply a warm, wet towel around your throat. Change it frequently. When you shower, point the warm water at your throat for one minute.

* Breathe through your nose, not your mouth.

WHAT SHOULDN'T YOU DO?

* Avoid spicy and fried food. Don't eat raw or cold food.
* Don't smoke, as it dries your throat.

Food Therapy

* Gargle green tea with honey:

   Ingredients: Green tea (Woo Lon, for example), honey.

   Procedure: Brew green tea with boiled water. Wait a few minutes, add 1 Tbs. of honey. Stir well. When the temperature goes down, vigorously gargle.

* Drink water chestnut juice. Peel water chestnuts. Place them in a juicer to make juice and drink often.

* Eat Asian pear with herb:

   Ingredients: 1 Asian pear, 1/8 oz. thunbery fritillary bulb powder (available in Chinese herb stores), 30 ml honey.

   Procedure: Take the center of the pear out and fill with thunbery fritillary bulb powder. Place the pear in a bowl and add honey. Steam it until well done. Divide it into two portions. Eat one portion twice a day.

* Take egg with sesame oil and sugar:

   Ingredients: 1 egg, 1 tsp. sesame oil, 1/2 tsp. sugar.

   Procedure: Beat an egg with sesame oil and sugar. Pour the mixture into a pan with 1 cup of boiling water on the stove. Cook for 40 seconds. Drink twice a day.

Chinese Herbs

 ☙ Squirt the patent herb Shuang Liao Hou Feng San into
   your throat.
 ☙ Drink boat sterculia seed tea:

   Ingredients: 5 boat sterculia seeds.

   Procedure: Place seeds in a pot and add 3 cups of water. Bring to a boil. Reduce heat and simmer for five
   minutes. The seeds will become very puffy. Remove
   the seeds and drink the decoction as tea frequently.

Low Blood Pressure

WHAT IS IT AND WHAT CAUSES IT?

If your blood pressure is below 90/60, that is considered low blood
pressure or hypotension. Normal blood pressure is around 120/80.
The symptoms of low blood pressure are often light-headedness, fatigue, or headaches. Orthostatic hypotension is a dangerous type of
low blood pressure. It happens when suddenly standing up from sitting or lying down. Along with arteriosclerosis, hypotension can be
caused by some medications, diabetes, or hormone disorders.

WHEN SHOULD YOU SEE A DOCTOR?

Sudden low blood pressure sometimes means that you may have a
fatal situation. You should go to an emergency room. If you have
chronic low blood pressure, see a doctor.

WHAT SHOULD YOU DO IN DAILY LIFE?

 ☙ Maintain good nutrition. Eat more lamb, pepper, ginger,
   Chinese chive, beans, or spicy food. Take in enough salt
   in your diet.
 ☙ Drink plenty of water. Drink coffee or tea.
 ☙ Frequent short, warm baths may help.
 ☙ Rest and get enough sleep. Overexertion makes blood
   pressure lower.

- If you feel dizzy when you get up, follow the next three steps:
  - Keep lying in bed for 30 seconds. Meanwhile, try to move your limbs, rub your face, and knead your abdomen.
  - Change to a sitting position for 30 seconds.
  - Finally, slowly get off the bed to stand up.
- Exercise regularly by walking, jogging, or doing Tai Chi. Increase your workload gradually.
- Promptly treat the underlying disease, which can lead to low blood pressure.

WHAT SHOULDN'T YOU DO?

- Don't miss your breakfast. It might be the reason for your low blood pressure.
- Don't eat celery, winter melon, red small beans, and hawthorn.
- Avoid physically demanding activities and climbing to a high altitude. Avoid standing for a long time or changing your body position too much.

Folk Remedies

- Alternately taking cold and warm baths may solve your problem. Prepare two buckets, one with warm water about 104 degrees Fahrenheit, and the other with cold water about 68 degrees Fahrenheit. Soak your arms or legs in the warm water for one minute. Then soak in cold water for 30 seconds. Repeat five times. Soak your arms or legs in warm water to finish.
- The following recipes may help you:
  - Drink strong tea and eat pickles frequently.
  - Eat 10 pieces of red dates twice a day.
  - Eat five cloves of walnuts at a time three times a day.
  - Eat 1/4 oz. longan aril a day, which is available in Chinese grocery stores.
  - Add ginger to your diet.

Food Therapy

🌿 Drink lycium fruit wine:

> **Ingredients:** 3 oz. lycium fruit, 5 oz. sugar, 750 ml 80-proof vodka.
>
> **Procedure:** Soak lycium and sugar in vodka for two months in a cold room (not in a refrigerator). It will become thick and sticky. Drink 20 ml herbal vodka with 30 ml water before bedtime.

🌿 Eat chicken with pineapple:

> **Ingredients:** 10 oz. fresh pineapple, 3 oz. chicken breast, salt, cooking oil.
>
> **Procedure:** Slice pineapple and chicken. Stir-fry with cooking oil until well done. Add salt. Eat every other day.

Chinese Massage

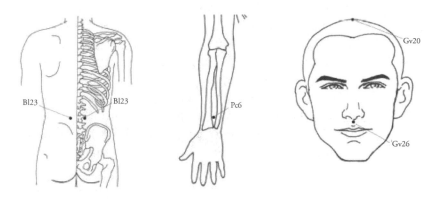

🌿 In acute cases, use the tip of the thumb to press the groove below the nose, slightly more than halfway up (Gv26). Press the point two thumb-widths above the wrist crease of the palm side, between the tendons, right under the buckle of the watchstrap (Pc6).

☞ Use the tip of your thumb to gently press the point right on the top crown center of your head, on the line connecting the earlobes for 30 seconds (Gv20). Then use the middle finger to gently press and knead the same point for one minute.

☞ Use the knuckles of both hands to gently press and knead the points a little higher than the waist, two finger-widths on both sides of the spine for one minute (Bl23).

☞ Use both your palms to scrub and knead the sacral bone area on the midline of your body on the back for one minute.

Chinese Herbs

☞ Take the patent herb Bu Zhong Yi Qi Wan. Follow the instructions.

☞ Eat chicken with herbs:

Ingredients: 1 hen, 1/2 oz. astragalus root, 1/4 oz. gastrodia tuber, 1/4 oz. green onion, 1/4 oz. ginger, 10 ml Chinese cooking wine, 1/4 oz. tangerine peels, salt.

Procedure: Soak the hen in boiled water for two minutes. Wrap herbs with gauze, place them inside the hen and place hen in a pot. Add green onion, ginger salt, wine, tangerine peels, and water to cover all ingredients. Turn on low heat and cook until done. Discard the herbs. Add some pepper and divide into three portions. Eat one portion a day for three days.

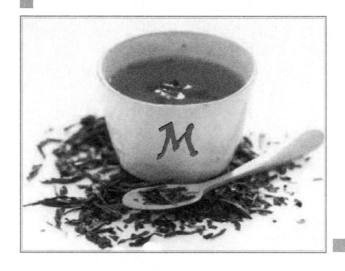

Meniere's Disease

WHAT IS IT AND WHAT CAUSES IT?

Meniere's disease is an inner ear disorder. The symptoms are vertigo, ringing in the ears, dizziness, nausea, and vomiting. Too much fluid in the membranous labyrinth is the main cause of Meniere's disease.

WHEN SHOULD YOU SEE A DOCTOR?

If you have persistent dizziness, ringing in the ears, or hearing loss, call your doctor.

WHAT SHOULD YOU DO IN DAILY LIFE?

- To lie down and rest is the first choice. If you need to move, do it very slowly.
- Control the intake of salt. Eat more winter melon, taro root, red small beans, and pearl barley.
- Take it easy. Exhaustion, anger, arguments, and dangerous, tense activities are the triggers.

WHAT SHOULDN'T YOU DO?

- When an attack comes, avoid any big visual or acoustic stimulation. Keep your room quiet and not too bright. Avoid sudden movement of the head and neck. Don't bend your back unless it is necessary.

- Don't drink water more than necessary. Drink less coffee and tea.

- Avoid spicy, greasy, raw, and cold food. Don't eat lamb, sea fish, and milk, which may trigger an attack.

- Don't come into contact with a chemical solution such as paint cleaner.

- Don't drink alcohol at all. Don't smoke.

Folk Remedies

- Eat eggs with herbs:

    Ingredients: 1 oz. pubescent angelica root, 6 eggs.

    Procedure: Add 3 cups of water and cook the ingredients for five minutes. Shell the eggs. Use a knife to cut several narrow openings in each egg. Place eggs back in the pot. Simmer for another 15 minutes. Discard the herbs and liquid. Eat two eggs at a time, once a day, for three days.

- Drink sunflower petal tea:

    Ingredients: 4 oz. sunflower petal (dried, without seeds), 2 Tbs. sugar.

    Procedure: Wash the petals clean. Cut into small pieces and put in a pot with 4 cups of water. Bring to a boil. Reduce heat and simmer for 15 minutes. Strain the decoction into a container. Then start a second batch. Add 2 cups of water into the pot and follow the above instructions to make another decoction. Mix the two decoctions together. The decoction is light brown. Add sugar, and drink 100 ml one hour after meals, twice a day for seven days. Keep unused decoction in the refrigerator.

Chinese Massage

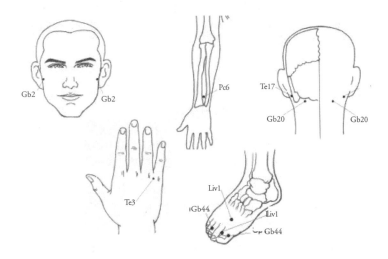

- ☞ Cover both ears with your hands and place the tip of the index and middle fingers on the point in the depression at the bottom of the skull, outside of the two big muscles on the neck, which you can feel by bending your neck forward and your head down (Gb20). Use the tips rhythmically to tap against that place for one minute.

- ☞ Use your thumb to gently press the point between the big toe and second toe, two finger-widths up the foot from the web between the toes for three minutes (Liv3).

- ☞ Use your thumb to gently press and knead the depression directly behind the earlobe on both sides for one minute (Te17).

- ☞ Use the tip of your thumb to gently press the point two thumb-widths above the wrist crease of the palm side, between the tendons, right under the buckle of the watchstrap (Pc6). Gradually increase the force until you feel a sensation of soreness and fullness.

- ☞ Use your thumb to knead the point in front of the ear, in the hollow formed as the mouth is open, for one minute (Gb2).

☞ Use your thumb to gently press the point between the ring and little fingers in the depression right below the two knuckles on the back of the hand (Te3). Gently press and knead for five to seven seconds. Meanwhile, inhale first, and then exhale slowly. Switch hands to do the same. Repeat five times.

Heat Therapy

Light a smokeless moxa stick first, which is like a cigar. Circle it one to two inches above the following points on both feet for five minutes. Do it one to two times a day. Be careful not to let the stick or its ashes burn you. You can use a cigarette instead of a moxa stick.

☞ The midpoint right above the base of the big toenail.

☞ The point on the big toe at the little toe side of the corner of the toenail. (Liv1)

☞ The point at the baseline and inner corner of the big toenail (Sp1).

☞ The point at the outside edge of the fourth toe, at the corner of the baseline of the toenail (Gb44).

Chinese Herbs

☞ If you have frequent vertigo, severe ear ringing, hearing loss, nausea, vomiting, or sore back and limbs, take the patent herb Liu Wei Di Huang Wan. Follow the instructions.

☞ If you often have a sudden vertigo attack with a fear of opening your eyes, nausea, or vomiting, take the patent herb Er Chen Wan. Follow the instructions.

Menopause

WHAT IS IT AND WHAT CAUSES IT?

It is the transitional process during which a woman stops menstruating. Though it's natural, in some women, menopause brings along terrible discomforts caused by decreased production of the hormones estrogen and progesterone. The symptoms are irregular periods, hot flashes, sweating, depression or anxiety, and dryness of the vagina.

WHEN SHOULD YOU SEE A DOCTOR?

If you experience menopause-related discomforts or unexplained bleeding, you should see your doctor to make sure you don't have any other medical conditions.

WHAT SHOULD YOU DO IN DAILY LIFE?

- ✷ Understand that menopause is an individual process that every woman goes through.
- ✷ Eat more bean products, dates, lily bulbs, walnuts, lotus seeds, dry mushrooms, and vegetables.
- ✷ Aerobic exercise is very important. You should get the equivalent of 30 minutes of fast walking every day. Research shows that exercise can boost the level of chemicals, such as serotonin, that regulate mood, and therefore uplift your spirits.
- ✷ Sex may have a positive effect on the symptoms (a personal lubricant may be necessary).

WHAT SHOULDN'T YOU DO?

- ✷ Avoid spicy food, alcohol, coffee, and other overstimulating substances. During menopause, these substances can trigger hot flashes or aggravate existing hot flash episodes. Don't eat foods that have a high-salt content as this increases the chance of edema.
- ✷ Don't tell your family or friends you are okay when they express concerns for your condition, if you are, in fact, miserable. If you don't let out your true feelings, your family may be less understanding of your symptoms, such as moodiness.

Food Therapy

- ☞ Every morning drink 1 cup of soymilk, which contains phytoestrogen.

☞ Drink egg soup with walnuts:

> **Ingredients:** 1 egg, 1/2 oz. walnuts, 1 Tbs. sugar.
>
> **Procedure:** Beat one egg. Crush walnuts into small pieces. Boil 1 cup of water. Pour the egg into the water and stir well. Add walnuts and sugar, and cook for 30 seconds. Drink once a day.

☞ Chop a half block of tofu into small pieces and put them into a pan. Add 1 cup of water and heat. After water is boiling, continue at low setting for another minute. Add some salt and soy sauce. Drink the soup once a day.

☞ Eat rice with nuts:

> **Ingredients:** 2 oz. red small beans, 10 red dates, 1 oz. walnuts, 1 oz. sticky rice.
>
> **Procedure:** Soak red beans in water overnight. Place all ingredients in a pot with 4 cups of water and bring to a boil. Reduce heat and simmer until mushy. Eat it once a day.

Chinese Massage

Massage once a day. Do not massage your abdomen and lower back during your period.

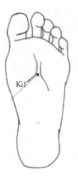 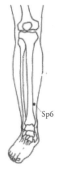 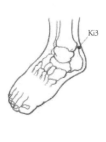

☞ Place your right palm on your abdomen and overlap with the left palm. Gently rub clockwise for one minute.

Place your palms on each side of the abdomen, and scrub horizontally toward the other side for one minute.

☞ Use both palms to scrub your lower back for one minute. Start from where you can reach and massage down to the sacrum.

☞ Use your thumb to gently press and knead the muscles on the back of your neck from top to bottom for one minute.

☞ Gently press the following points for one minute:

　☞ The point four finger-widths up from the inside anklebone, right behind the leg bone (Sp6).

　☞ The point below the ball of the foot in the center, about a third of the distance between the toes and the heel (Ki1).

　☞ The depression behind the top of the inside anklebone (Ki3).

Qi Gong

Do the following step by step:

☞ Stand naturally with feet shoulder width apart and arms hanging by the sides. Keep breathing naturally and slowly. Hold a relaxed countenance on your face.

☞ Once you are relaxed, inhale deeply through your nose. When breathing in, gradually raise your buttocks, shoulders, and head along with heels. Your chest will stretch naturally and your abdomen will gradually fill. When your lungs are almost filled, draw back your shoulder blades and breathe in even deeper. Then breathe out slowly and bring your heels back to the ground slowly. Your belly will naturally deflate. Repeat this breathing sequence eight times and then return to the original stance.

☞ Following the previous sequence, relax all parts of your body with your mind. When breathing in, silently say, "Peace." When breathing out, silently say, "Relax." Repeat this procedure eight times.

- ☞ Slightly bend your knees, keeping a slight tension in the hips. Start to shake your body in a natural rhythm. Do so for two minutes, then slow down gradually and stop.
- ☞ Take a deep breath. Slightly bend your knees with arms naturally hanging by the sides. Slowly turn your body to the right. Slowly return to your initial position. Following the opposite pattern, start to turn your body to the left. Repeat this procedure (left and right) eight times.
- ☞ To finish, place your palms together and raise your arms above your head. Breathe out and at the same time slowly lower your arms level with your navel.

Chinese Herbs

- ☞ If you have hot flashes, sweating, irritability, warm sensations in your palms and soles, or red-colored menstrual flows, take the patent herb Zhi Bai Di Huang Wan. Follow the instructions.
- ☞ If you have an irregular period or no period for several months, light-colored menstrual flow with clots, cold limbs, loose stool, and an aversion to cold take the patent herb Jin Gui Shen Qi Wan. Follow the instructions.

Menstrual Problem 1: Absence of Periods (Amenorrhea)

WHAT IS IT AND WHAT CAUSES IT?

Amenorrhea is the medical term for the absence of periods. In Western medicine, this condition is divided into two types: If you are over 16 years old, but never had menstruation, you may have primary amenorrhea. If your periods have ceased for more than three months, then you may have secondary amenorrhea. The main causes of amenorrhea are hormonal problems, stopping the usage of birth control pills, obesity, excessive stress, rapid weight loss, or too much exercise.

WHEN SHOULD YOU SEE A DOCTOR?

When you have a menstrual problem, see a doctor to rule out other underlying disease (or pregnancy).

WHAT SHOULD YOU DO IN DAILY LIFE?

- ↳ Get an adequate amount of sleep.
- ↳ Nutrition is essential. Eat more eggs, lean meats, fish, milk, red dates, Chinese black fungus, orange, hawthorn fruit, peaches, and brown sugar.
- ↳ Exercise regularly.

WHAT SHOULDN'T YOU DO?

- ↳ Avoid stressful situations, and guard against both physical and mental exhaustion. An optimistic mind is very important to keep endocrine function working normally.
- ↳ Don't worry too much if you don't have a period after you change your lifestyle or move to a new place. It could be a normal body reaction.
- ↳ Don't eat too much salty and greasy food if you are already overweight. Control your weight.
- ↳ Avoid abortion if at all possible.
- ↳ If you are breastfeeding, don't continue longer than the necessary period.

Food Therapy

If you are over 16 years old and have not started your period yet, or menstrual flow gradually decreases to nothing, and you suffer from lethargy, dizziness, and weakness of limb, do the following:

- ☞ Take turtle soup:

    Ingredients: A whole turtle, 3 oz. lean pork, 1/4 oz. euconmmia bark, 1/4 oz. dang gui, 1/4 oz. cooked rehmannia.

    Procedure: Wash thoroughly. Wrap herbs in gauze. Cover all the ingredients with water in a pot and bring to a boil.

Reduce heat and simmer until the turtle is very soft. Discard the herbs and add salt. Divide into three portions. Eat one portion a day for three days.

If your menstrual schedule is gradually postponed, menstrual flow is small, and thin with light color and gradually stops, and you are tired, dizzy, and have heart palpitations, do the following:

☞ Eat lamb with herbs:

Ingredients: 1/4 oz. dang gui, 1/4 oz. astragulas, 1/4 oz. ginger, 5 oz. lamb.

Procedure: Slice ginger into small pieces. Cut lamb into small pieces. Wrap herbs in gauze. Cover all ingredients with water and cook until lamb is very soft. Discard the herbs and add salt. Eat lamb and drink soup once a day. Continue to take for five days each month.

If your period stops due to emotional stress, you have lower abdominal pain with a bloating sensation, and you are irritable, do the following:

☞ Take hawthorn with sugar:

Ingredients: 2 oz. hawthorn (without kernel), 1 oz. brown sugar.

Procedure: Place hawthorn in a pot. Add 3 cups of water and bring to a boil. Reduce heat and simmer for 20 minutes. Strain the decoction and add sugar. Divide into two portions. Drink twice a day on an empty stomach.

If you are overweight and have a bloating sensation in the chest, nausea, lots of phlegm, and exhaustion, you can do the following:

☞ Take pearl barley with herb:

Ingredients: 1/2 oz. dried white beans, 1 oz. Chinese pearl barley, 1/2 oz. hawthorn (these are available at Chinese grocery stores), 1 oz. brown sugar.

Procedure: Stir-fry white beans for two minutes on low heat. Place all ingredients in a pot and add 4 cups of water. Bring to a boil and simmer until they are soft. Eat once a day. Continue to take for seven days every month.

If your period suddenly stops, and you have lower abdominal pain that gets better with warmth, an aversion to cold, and loose stool, do the following:

- Drink dates with herbs:

    Ingredients: 1/4 oz. ligusticum, 1/4 oz. ginger, 30 red dates, 2 oz. brown sugar.

    Procedure: Soak the dates in water for three hours. Wrap the ligusticum with gauze. Place all the ingredients in a pot, add 2 cups of water, and bring to a boil. Simmer until the water is almost gone. Eat 10 dates at a time. Take three times a day for seven days each month.

Qi Gong

Do the following step by step:

- In the evening when the moon has just risen, stand facing the moon in a quiet place. Place your feet shoulder width apart. Place your tongue against the palate. Breathe naturally.
- Inhale and visualize the air going down to the region two finger-widths below your belly button. Hold your breath in for as long as possible. Then exhale. Repeat this process eight times.
- Raise your head toward the moon. Close your eyes a little bit (still open). Walk slowly toward the moon and breathe naturally. Imagine inhaling the essence of the moon, then bring it down to the region two finger-widths below the belly button. Slowly exhale. Repeat this 20 times.
- Return your head to normal position and close your eyes. Overlap your palms and place them on the point at two finger-widths below the belly button. Relax your whole body and stand quietly. Naturally breathe 20 times.

Chinese Massage

Massage once a day. Do not massage your lower abdomen and lower back when you are menstruating.

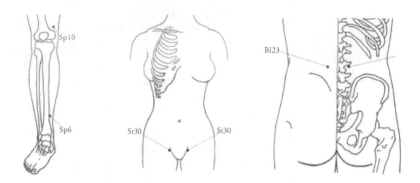

- ☞ Rub your hands against each other until warm. Place your right palm on your lower abdomen. Overlap with the left palm. Gently rub clockwise for three minutes.
- ☞ Gently press and knead the points a little higher than the waist, two finger-widths on both sides of the spine for two minutes (Bl23).
- ☞ Use the pad of your thumb to gently press the point just above the upper edge of the pubic bone and two thumb-widths on either side of the midline of the abdomen until your lower limbs feel warm (St30).
- ☞ Gently press and knead the following points for one minute:
  - ☞ The point four finger-widths up from the inside ankle-bone, right behind the leg bone (Sp6).
  - ☞ The point on the top of the inside edge of the knee. Flex your knee and place your hand on the kneecap. The point is where your thumb touches (Sp10). Gradually increase the pressure until you have a sensation of soreness and distention.

Menstrual Problem 2: Menstrual Cramps (Dysmenorrhea)

WHAT IS IT AND WHAT CAUSES IT?

During, prior to, or after menstruation, women have pain in the lower abdomen, lower back, or thigh regions, which are caused by the uterine muscles contracting. It is a result of excessive prostaglandin in your body during menstruation. It may be accompanied by headache, fatigue, and nausea. Secondary dysmenorrhea is caused by an underlying gynecological disorder, which needs to be treated first.

WHEN SHOULD YOU SEE A DOCTOR?

If you have severe pain, or pain that lasts more than two days, or if pain occurs between your periods, see a doctor.

WHAT SHOULD YOU DO IN DAILY LIFE?

* Take care of it before it starts. One week before your period, you should eat less fatty, and more fiber rich and easily digested food. Remember that spicy foods, alcohol, and coffee, will increase pain during your period.
* Have regular bowel movements.
* Take it easy. Nervousness is one of the trigger factors of dysmenorrhea.
* Sleep and get up on time. Poor lifestyle may contribute to dysmenorrhea.
* Aerobic exercise will improve blood circulation and provide some relief.

WHAT SHOULDN'T YOU DO?

* Don't expose yourself to cold during your period. Don't swim. Don't eat cold foods such as ice cream.
* Don't wear high heel shoes, which may cause dysmenorrhea.
* Don't have sex during your period.

* Don't take painkillers without consulting your doctor during your period.

Folk Remedies

* Dip a cotton ball into 70-percent rubbing alcohol and squeeze out excess alcohol. Insert it in your ear for 30 minutes. If you have an allergic reaction, discontinue use.

* Apply the patent herb Tiger Balm on your belly button, two or three times a day. If you have an allergic reaction, discontinue use.

* Apply salt with ginger and green onion:

    Ingredients: 4 oz. fresh ginger, 2 oz. green onion, 1 lb. salt.

    Procedure: Thinly slice the ginger and green onion stalk, and mix with salt and stir-fry five minutes on medium heat. Wrap the herbs in a towel and apply to the painful spot while still warm. Be careful not to burn yourself.

* Take a warm bath. While in the tub, gently tap your soles and both sides of the feet with a hairbrush for five minutes. The hairbrush acts like a bunch of acupuncture needles to stimulate the meridian and prompt the circulation of Qi and blood. Use your finger to gently press and knead the second toe and the area on the inside of the ankle directly below the anklebone.

Food Therapy

* Drink black tea with sugar:

    Ingredients: 1 Tbs. black tea leaves, 1 Tbs. brown sugar.

    Procedure: Use boiled water to brew the tea for five minutes. Add sugar and drink after each meal, three times a day. Start five days before your period, and stop when the menstrual flow starts.

* Drink salvia vodka:

    Ingredients: 500 ml 80-proof vodka, 2 oz. salvia (available in Chinese herb stores).

Procedure: Soak salvia and vodka in a sealed bottle for one month. Discard the herb. Drink 15 ml of this mixture with 20 ml water, two times a day. Start one week before your period, and stop when the period comes.

Heat Therapy

☞ Warm up two potatoes. Use them to gently press and roll over your lower abdominal area for five minutes. Start three days before the period, twice a day. Stop when the period comes.

☞ Light a smokeless moxa stick, which is like a cigar. Circle it one to two inches above the following areas for 10 minutes, one or two times a day. Be careful to not let the stick or its ashes burn you.

   ☞ *Lower abdomen:* on the midline four finger-widths below the belly button (Cv4).

   ☞ *Lower abdomen:* the point two thumb-widths on either side of the midline of the abdomen and a hand-width under the belly button (St29).

   ☞ *Leg:* The depression four finger-widths below the knee-cap edge and one thumb's-width outside of the shin-bone (St36).

   ☞ *Leg:* The point four finger-widths up from the inside anklebone, right behind the leg bone (Sp6).

Chinese Massage

Start your massage seven days before your period. Don't massage your abdomen and lower back area when your period begins.

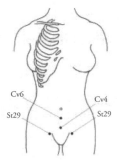

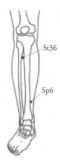

☞ Rub your palms against each other until they are warm. Rub your lower abdomen clockwise for two minutes. Use the heel of your palm to push your bellybutton down for two minutes.

☞ Use your middle finger to gently press and knead the point four finger-widths below your bellybutton on the middle of the abdomen for two minutes (Cv4).

☞ Tap and scrub the lumbar region for two minutes.

☞ Gently press the depression four finger-widths below the kneecap edge and one thumb's-width outside of the shin-bone (St36).

☞ Gently press and knead the point four finger-widths up from the inside anklebone, right behind the leg bone for one minute (Sp6).

Qi Gong

☞ Lie down in a quiet room. Drink a little warm water. Loosen your clothes and belt. Mentally and physically relax.

☞ Silently repeat a phrase such as, "Cramping go away," with breathing. Inhale while silently saying, "Cramping." Hold the breath while silently saying, "go." Exhale while silently saying the last word, "away." Continue to do silently for five minutes.

☞ Do belly breathing: When inhaling, raise the tongue against the hard palate, which naturally conducts Qi to the lower abdomen. Imagine the Qi sinking to the point below the bellybutton. When exhaling, detach the tongue from the hard palate so the breath can exit naturally.

Chinese Herbs

Generally, you can take the patent herb Yun Nan Bai Yao. Follow the instructions.

Therea are four types of dysmenorrhea in Chinese medicine.

If you have distending pain and tenderness before or during period, which is worse with pressure, a small menstrual flow with dark-red color and clots, and some relief after discharge of clots, do the following:

> ☞ Take the patent herb Chai Hu Shu Gan Wan. Follow the instructions.

Chinese Herbs

> ☞ Eat eggs cooked with herbs:
>
> **Ingredients:** 2 eggs, 1/4 oz. ligusticum, 2 Tbs. Chinese cooking wine.
>
> **Procedure:** Add 2 cups of water and cook eggs with the herbs until the eggs are well done. Peel the shell and slice a few cuts on the eggs. Add cooking wine to water and cook another three minutes. Remove the residue of the herbs. Eat the eggs and drink the decoction once a day for five to seven days. Start three days before your period.

If you have distending pain with a heavy sensation and a sensation of squeezing before or during your period, which becomes worse with pressure, and is better with warmth; a small dark menstrual flow with clots; and coldness of limbs, do the following:

> ☞ Take the patent herb Tong Jing Wan. Follow the instructions.
>
> ☞ Eat red dates with dried ginger:
>
> **Ingredients:** 1/2 oz. red dates, 1/2 oz. dried ginger, 1/4 oz. prickly-ash peel.
>
> **Procedure:** First add 1 cup of water to the dates and ginger and bring to a boil. Add prickly ash peels and continue to simmer for 10 minutes on low heat. Drink the decoction and eat the dates once a day for five days. Start three days before the period.

If you have pain with hot sensations before your period, which is worse with pressure, thick menstrual flow with dark-red color and clots, and a thick and yellow discharge, do the following:

> ☞ Take the patent herb Er Miao Wan. Follow the instructions.

❧ Drink red small bean, pearl barley, and rice soup:

Ingredients: 2 oz. red small beans, 1 oz. Chinese pearl barley, 3 oz. rice.

Procedure: Soak red beans and pearl barley in water overnight. Add 4 cups of water with all ingredients to make rice soup. Drink twice a day. Start seven days before your period.

If you have vague pain with a dragging feeling before or after your period, which can be alleviated by warmth or pressure, a small thin menstrual flow with light color, and a lack of vitality, do the following:

❧ Take the patent herb Wu Ji Bai Feng Wan. Follow the instructions.

❧ Eat red dates and longan aril with herbs:

Ingredients: 3 oz. red dates, 1 oz. longan aril (a kind of Asian fruit), 1 oz. dang gui, 2 eggs.

Procedure: Soak the dates in water for three hours. Add 3 cups of water to the herbs, and bring to a boil. Reduce heat and simmer for 20 minutes. Break 2 eggs into the decoction, and cook for another minute. Discard the dang gui residue only. Drink the decoction once a day for five days. Start three days before your period.

Menstrual Problem 3: Premenstrual Syndrome

WHAT IS IT AND WHAT CAUSES IT?

Premenstrual syndrome is a condition caused by a hormonal imbalance one or two weeks before every period. Some of the symptoms include a headache, dizziness, edema, acne, bloating, irritability, and depression. (For **Menstrual Cramps**, see page 213.)

WHEN SHOULD YOU SEE A DOCTOR?

If the symptoms are too debilitating and not responding to self-treatment, call a doctor.

WHAT SHOULD YOU DO IN DAILY LIFE?

- Control your emotions: Take it easy. Always having optimistic, positive attitudes will help you in the menstrual period. When you are feeling moodiness and anger swelling up, take a deep breath and tell yourself to calm down.
- Tell your family, especially your spouse, about your condition so they will understand. It can help to ease the tension and conflict during PMS.
- Be sure to get adequate exercise, such as walking for 30 minutes a day.
- Eat more vegetables and fruits. Control the intake of salt.

WHAT SHOULDN'T YOU DO?

- Don't consume too much overstimulatory items such as caffeine, alcohol, excessive salt, and refined sugar. Chinese medicine thinks most cases of PMS have fire. These foods bring fire in your body.
- Avoid any stressful situations when anticipating the symptoms of PMS. Do things that make you happy and avoid activities that will irritate you.

Folk Remedies

- Start five days before your period. Use a plastic bottle filled with warm water as hot as you feel comfortable and roll over it on your lower abdomen for 15 minutes. Stop when the period comes.
- Apply fennel fruit with cinnamon powder:
  Ingredients: 1 oz. fennel fruit, 1/2 oz. cinnamon powder.
  Procedure: Stir-fry all ingredients to warm in a pan on low heat. Place in a cotton bag and apply on your belly button for 30 minutes, once a day. Start three days before your period and stop when it comes.

Food Therapy

- If you have a sensation of fullness and soreness in your breasts, and a heavy sensation in the lower abdomen, eat more celery, kelp, black beans, winter melon, watermelon, pork, and beef.

☞ If you have a headache, insomnia, irritability, or general lassitude, eat more lily bulb, longan aril, lotus seeds, dates, and honey. They are available in Chinese grocery stores.

☞ Eat black beans and eggs with rice wine:

Ingredients: 2 eggs, 2 oz. black beans, 120 ml rice wine.

Procedure: Soak beans in water overnight. Add 2 cups of water in a pot with the eggs and beans. Cook until beans are soft. Take eggshells off. Continue to cook for one minute. Pour the rice wine in the pot. Eat eggs and drink the soup once a day. Start five days before your period and stop when the period comes.

Chinese Massage

Don't massage your abdomen or lower back during your period.

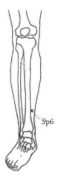
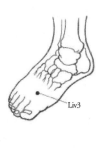

☞ Rub your palms against each other until they become warm. Place both hands on your lower back in the sacrum area. Push and scrub from bottom up until you have a warm sensation.

☞ Place your palms on your upper abdomen. Rub gently clockwise from top down to your lower abdomen.

☞ Place both your hands on top of your head. Use your fingertips to gently tap downward toward your forehead, then tap back through top. Continue to tap backwards along the midline down to your neck. Change the direction again, tapping upward to the vertex (top) of your head. Repeat five times. Finally, use your palms to gently rub and knead the vertex for 30 seconds.

☙ Gently press and knead the point four finger-widths up from the inside anklebone, right behind the leg bone (Sp6).

☙ Gently press the point between the big toe and second toe, two finger-widths up the foot from the web between the toes for one minute (Liv3).

☙ Place both hands below your kneecaps, the thumb inside and the four fingers outside. Push down to your ankles three times. Place your hand on the calf and push down to the ankles three times.

Chinese Herbs

☙ Take the patent herb Dan Zhi Xiao Yao Wan. Follow the instructions.

Menstrual Problem 4: Uterine Bleeding (Dysfunctional)

WHAT IS IT AND WHAT CAUSES IT?

Dysfunctional uterine bleeding is irregular and unpredictable vaginal bleeding. The condition is usually caused by a hormonal imbalance associated with stress or major developmental stages of life, such as puberty and menopause.

Heavy periods are a type of dysfunctional uterine bleeding, and in this book we will focus on this type. People who suffer from it would have bleeding that feels like gushing, and also the bleeding days may last much longer than the days of a normal period.

WHEN SHOULD YOU SEE A DOCTOR?

If you are losing a lot of blood and are unable to stop it, you should immediately seek professional medical attention. If your periods are irregular, especially when the bleedings are small and continuous, see the doctor early to prevent the condition from developing further.

WHAT SHOULD YOU DO IN DAILY LIFE?

- When your period is heavy, get bed rest. Prop up the upper part of your body to facilitate the flow of menses.
- Control your emotions: Anger, depression, or other upsets will cause irregularity of your menstruation. Maintaining a confident and positive attitude is key.
- Maintain a diet of diverse nutrients.
- Keep good hygiene of the genital area. Shower instead of bathing.

WHAT SHOULDN'T YOU DO?

- Do not take baths. When bleeding is heavy, avoid taking hot showers to prevent heightened circulation, which would result in even heavier bleeding.
- Don't drink alcohol, and don't eat spicy foods such as onions, hot pepper, or mustard.
- Avoid overexertion and excessive tension.
- Don't have sex during this time.

Folk Remedies

- When the bleeding is heavy, take a lighted moxa stick (available in Chinese herb stores—you can also use incense) and hold it above the point at the baseline and inner corner of the big toenail (Sp1). Let it hover near enough to feel warmth. Do so on both toes for a half hour each time, two or three times a day. When the bleeding is getting better, reduce it to once a day. (Take care not to burn yourself.)
- Inhale rice vinegar steam to stop bleeding: Find two white baseball-size stones. Put in a fireplace and heat until they are red. Place one of them in a metal container with 500 ml rice vinegar. Inhale the vinegar steam for 20 minutes. When the stone cools change to the other one.

Food Therapy

☞ If you have anemia, drink date soup:

Ingredients: 7 dates, 7 dried litchis (available in Chinese grocery stores).

Procedure: Add ingredients and 2 cups of water to a pot and cook for five minutes to make soup. Drink once a day.

☞ If you have poor appetite, drink lotus seed soup:

Ingredients: 2 oz. lotus seeds, 1 oz. rice, sugar.

Procedure: Take the inner sprout of lotus seeds out. Soak the lotus seeds in water overnight. Add 3 cups of water and all ingredients to a pot and bring to a boil. Reduce heat and simmer for 30 minutes. Add sugar and eat once a day.

☞ If you have an aversion to cold, eat egg with herb:

Ingredients: 1/32 oz. deer pilose antler (available in Chinese herb stores), 1 egg.

Procedure: Beat the egg with 1/2 cup of water. Mix with pilose antler in a bowl. Steam for 15 minutes. Eat all once a day for one month.

☞ If you have an aversion to heat, drink fungus soup:

Ingredients: 1/4 oz. Chinese black fungus, 1/4 oz. Chinese white fungus, 1/2 oz. crystal sugar. They are available in Chinese grocery stores.

Procedure: Soak fungus in warm water for two hours. Wash them clean. Place them in a bowl with sugar and 1 cup of water. Steam for one hour. Divide into two portions. Eat once a day frequently.

Chinese Massage

Massage the following points once a day. Don't massage your abdomen and lower back during your period.

☞ Rub your hands against each other until warm. Use your right palm to rub the lower abdomen clockwise for three minutes.

☞ Gently press and knead the following points for one minute:

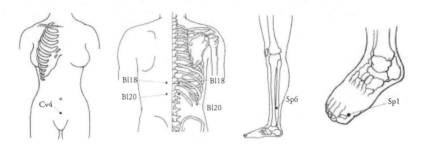

☞ The point on the midline of the abdomen four finger-widths below the belly button (Cv4).

☞ The point four finger-widths up from the inside ankle-bone, right behind the leg bone (Sp6).

☞ The point on the baseline and inner corner of the big toenail (Sp1).

☞ Make fists and use the knuckles to scrub the points located two finger-widths on both side of the spine, in your middle back (Bl18, Bl20).

Chinese Herbs

Take the following only when you *don't* have a period.

☞ Eat chicken with herb:
 Ingredients: One whole chicken, 1/2 oz. mugwort leaves, 60 ml rice wine.
 Procedure: Wrap the herb with gauze. Add water to cover all ingredients and cook until well done. Add salt and divide into three portions. Eat on alternate days for six days.

☞ Eat rice with herbs:
 Ingredients: 1 oz. donkey-hide gelatin, 3 oz. sticky rice.

Procedure: Add rice to 3 cups of water and make rice soup. At the last minute add crushed donkey gelatin and bring to a boil again. Cook until the gelatin is melted. Divide into two portions. Take twice a day for three days.

Motion Sickness

WHAT IS IT AND WHAT CAUSES IT?

Motion sickness is dizziness, nausea, vomiting, or other uneasiness caused by the temporary super sensitivity of the inner ear's balancing system. It happens while you are in a moving car, airplane, and boat.

WHEN SHOULD YOU SEE A DOCTOR?

If you travel a lot and this is a frequent problem, see a doctor.

WHAT SHOULD YOU DO IN DAILY LIFE?

- Rest before traveling.
- Sit in the front seat of a car. Find a cabin in the center of the ship, where the motion is at a minimum.
- Set your sight on something stationary. Focus on the road ahead or the horizon. Keep your head still. Don't read.
- Get fresh air. Open the window of the car, or go to the deck of the boat.

WHAT SHOULDN'T YOU DO?

- Before traveling don't eat too much. Don't travel with an empty stomach. Don't drink too much alcohol or carbonated soft drinks.

Folk Remedies

- Apply a piece of ginger at the point two thumb-widths above the wrist crease of the palm side, between the tendons, right under the buckle of the watchstrap (Pc6).

If you have an allergic reaction, discontinue use. Or place a mung bean at that point and affix with tape. Gently press this bean frequently.

☞ Apply a big piece of ginger to your belly button (navel) and cover it with tape. If you have an allergic reaction, discontinue use.

Food Therapy

☞ Thirty minutes before boarding, chew on a piece of ginger and spit out the residue, or eat 1/2 tsp. of ginger powder.

☞ During the trip, eating a few olives, a lemon, or crackers may help.

Chinese Massage

If you feel uncomfortable during the trip, choose the following and massage slowly:

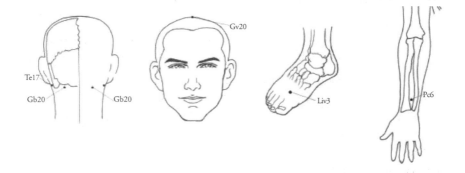

☞ Gently press the point in the depression directly behind the earlobe (Te17).

☞ Gently press and knead your temples.

☞ Gently press and knead the point in the depression at the bottom of the skull, outside of the two big muscles on the neck, which you can feel by bending down your neck (Gb20).

☞ Use your palm to gently pat and knead the center on top of your head, on the line connecting the two tips of your ears (Gv20).

☞ Gently press the point two thumb-widths above the wrist crease of the palm side, between the tendons, right under the buckle of the watchstrap (Pc6).

☞ Gently press the point between the big toe and second toe, two finger-widths up the foot from the web between the toes (Liv3).

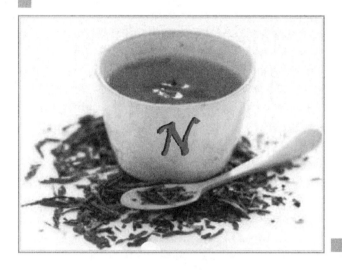

Neck Pain (Chronic)

WHAT IS IT AND WHAT CAUSES IT?

Neck pain can be divided into two categories:

- ❧ Neck pain, neck spasms, or stiffness. The cause is holding the head in an awkward position too long.
- ❧ Cervical spondylosis or cervical osteoarthritis. It is a common problem among the middle aged and elderly. The symptoms are pain, numbness, or stiffness in the head, neck, or shoulder. In severe cases, there may be unbearable pain, and an inability to rotate and bend upward. It is mostly caused by vertebrae degeneration, or calcification in the neck.

WHEN SHOULD YOU SEE A DOCTOR?

If you have sudden neck pain, see a doctor. If you have persistent neck pain, or no sign of improvement after you treat yourself, see a doctor.

WHAT SHOULD YOU DO IN DAILY LIFE?

- Sit in a firm chair with good back support and either keep the correct posture, or find something to support your lower back. Hold your head level as much as you can when you are working or resting. When you are chatting with someone, reverse your chair and place both forearms on the back support to relax your neck muscles.

- Sleep on a firm mattress and use the right pillow. Don't sleep on your stomach.

- Applying a hot water bottle to the neck may give you some relief. You can also apply a steamed warm towel around your neck and blow a low-power hair dryer on the area to keep a consistent temperature. Take care not to burn yourself.

- Taking vitamin C, vitamin E, and glucosamine chondroitin sulfate daily may help over the long term.

- **If your neck pain is caused by cervical spondylosis, you need to consult with your doctor first regarding neck exercise.** Otherwise, you can do the following neck exercises to prevent neck pain. These kinds of exercises change the normal moving direction of the shoulder and neck in daily life, and could alleviate the growth of a bone spur and give some pain relief.
  - Do a skipping rope exercise without rope. Jump with the tips of both feet. Rotate your arms forward 30 times, then backwards 30 times. *If you are elderly, don't use this method.*
  - Shrug both of your shoulders for five minutes in the morning.

WHAT SHOULDN'T YOU DO?

- Avoid exposure to cold and wet conditions. Always keep your neck warm for good circulation. Wear a shirt or pajamas with a collar, even in the summer.

- Avoid work with a tilted head for long periods, taking a rest between such work. Adjust the height of your desk to be a little higher.

❧ When you drive or somebody calls you from behind, don't turn your head very quickly. When you want to lift a heavy object, don't use only your arms. Instead use the whole body. These will help you to avoid local soft-tissue injuries in the neck.

❧ Don't wear high heel shoes.

Folk Remedies

❧ In a chronic case, rub liquor on the neck. Pour 4 Tbs. of liquor into a small metal container. Set it on fire to make it hot. Cover a lid to put out the flame. Dip a cotton ball into the liquor, then rub your neck once a day for three days. If you have an allergic reaction, discontinue use.

❧ Apply tofu with vinegar:

Ingredients: tofu, rice vinegar.

Procedure: Cut a 1/4-inch slice of tofu and use a fork to punch a lot of holes. In acute cases freeze the tofu in a refrigerator for five minutes. Soak it in a bowl with vinegar. Apply to the painful area for 15 minutes. In chronic cases, use a microwave to warm the tofu and apply to the painful area for 20 minutes. Reheat the tofu if necessary. If you have an allergic skin reaction, discontinue use.

❧ In a chronic case, apply hot salt with black beans and vinegar:

Ingredients: 3 oz. black beans, 2 lb. salt, 300 ml rice vinegar.

Procedure: Stir-fry the beans for three minutes on low heat. Grind them into small pieces. Mix with salt and stir-fry another five minutes. Add vinegar and stir well. Put in a cotton fabric bag. Apply to the painful spot once a day. Don't burn yourself.

Food Therapy

❧ If your pain moves around and is worse in a damp or cold condition, drink this herb soup:

Ingredients: 1 oz. Chinese pearl barley, 1/8 oz. cinnamon twig, 1/4 oz. ginger, 3 oz. rice.

Procedure: Place cinnamon twig and ginger in a pot. Add 1 cup of water and bring to a boil. Reduce heat and simmer for 10 minutes. Strain the decoction. Add 2 cups of water into the decoction. Add the barley and rice and continueto cook to make rice soup. Drink twice a day.

☛ If you have a fixed stitching pain, which is worse at night, drink Chinese rose tea:

Ingredients: 1/2 oz. fresh Chinese rose flower.

Procedure: Brew with boiled water and drink as tea.

Chinese Massage

Massage the following points once a day. You may need to ask your family member to help.

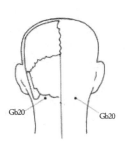
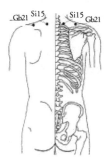
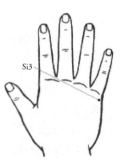

☛ Find the painful spot on your neck. Gently press and knead that spot.

☛ Move the index, middle, and ring fingers of both hands along the muscles beside the spine to find any pain point or hard node. Gently press and knead these spots.

☛ Gently press and knead the point in the depression at the bottom of the skull, outside of the two big muscles on the neck, which you can feel by bending your neck forward, head down, until you have a sensation of soreness and distention (Gb20). Use both hands to grasp the muscles from these two points down to both shoulders.

☞ Tap the points under the earlobes, right at the top of the shoulders (Gb21).

☞ Gently press and knead the point at two thumb-widths from the big bone at the base of the neck on either side of the spine (Si15).

☞ Gently press and knead the point on the side of your hand, just below the little finger joint at the end of the crease (Si3).

Chinese Herbs

☞ Apply the herb patch Shang Shi Zhi Tong Gao. If you have an allergic reaction, discontinue use.

☞ Apply a heating patch with herb, called Chinese Moxibustion. Follow the instructions.

☞ If your pain moves around and is worse in damp or cold conditions, take the patent herb Gu Ci Wan. Follow the instructions.

☞ If you have a stitching pain at a fixed region, which is worse at night, take the patent herb Huo Lou Wan. Follow the instructions.

☞ If you have had a dull pain for a long time, accompanied with dizziness, weakness of the back and knee, and the symptoms are worse with exertion, take the patent herb Kang Gu Ci Zeng Sheng Wan. Follow the instructions.

Nose Bleeding

WHAT IS IT AND WHAT CAUSES IT?

Nosebleeds are from ruptured blood vessels inside the nose, mostly from the septum. It starts and stops spontaneously. Dry air and minor trauma are the main causes for nosebleeds.

WHEN SHOULD YOU SEE A DOCTOR?

If your nosebleed happens after a head injury, see a doctor. If you treat yourself for more than 10 minutes with no success, or your nosebleed comes from the back of the nose and drains through the throat, or your nose bleeding becomes quite frequent, see a doctor.

WHAT SHOULD YOU DO IN DAILY LIFE?

- Sit down. Tilt your head forward a little to avoid the blood backing into the airway. Use your mouth to breath. Use the thumb and index finger to pinch the soft part between the nose bridge and the nostrils for five to 10 minutes. Soak a towel in cold water, squeeze out the excess water, and apply to your forehead and nose area.
- Maintain adequate humidity in your home.
- If you have nosebleeds quite often, think about taking a multivitamin with iron and take enough Vitamin C.
- Treat the underlying disease first, such as high blood pressure or leukemia.

WHAT SHOULDN'T YOU DO?

- After the bleeding stops, don't pick your nose.
- Don't eat hot spicy food. Eat less chocolate, coffee, cocoa, oranges, and apricots.
- If you have nosebleeds quite often, don't take unnecessary aspirin.

Folk Remedies

- There are some alternative ways to stop nosebleeds:
  - Hook your middle fingers to each other and pull outward very hard. If your child is too young to do this on his or her own, you can use your own fingers to hook your child's middle finger and pull.
  - In most cases, the bleeding only occurs in one side of nose. Raise the opposite arm and tilt your head backward a little and keep still. The bleeding should stop. Continue to raise your arm for a while. If the bleeding

comes from both sides, raise both arms. Stretch your arms up against your ears.

☞ Close your four fingers together and dip them in cold water. Gently tap your forehead.

☞ If you always have nosebleeds at night or in the early morning, use a cotton swab to apply some sesame oil to your nostril before bedtime.

Food Therapy

☞ Eat egg whites and sugar (for children):

Ingredients: 2 egg whites, 1 oz. sugar.

Procedure: Beat the eggs. Use 1 cup of boiled water with sugar to brew it for three minutes. Eat at once, twice a day.

☞ Drink radish juice with sugar:

Ingredients: Daikon radish, sugar.

Procedure: Slice radish and use a juicer to make juice. Add sugar. Drink 50 ml at a time, three times a day for three days.

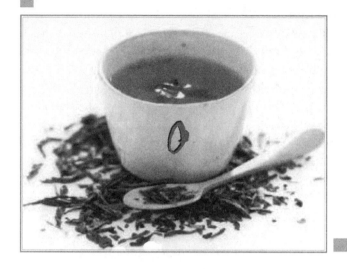

Osteoporosis

WHAT IS IT AND WHAT CAUSES IT?

Osteoporosis is a decreasing of the bone density marked by gradually losing height and becoming stooped. The symptoms include lower back pain, particularly when changing body positions or climbing stairs. In some cases there are no symptoms until a bone breaks. Women are more prone to get osteoporosis. After menopause, women have a lower level of estrogen which leads to increasing loss in bone density. Women also have smaller, lighter bones than men do, making them prone to losing bone mass sooner than men. Aging, lack of calcium, lack of physical activity, and genetics are the main causes of osteoporosis.

WHEN SHOULD YOU SEE A DOCTOR?

If you are older than age 65, you should have a bone-density test. If you have sudden pain, you should see a doctor to rule out a bone fracture. If you are a menopausal woman with a family history of osteoporosis, you should be tested as soon as possible.

WHAT SHOULD YOU DO IN DAILY LIFE?

» Take enough calcium with vitamin D before bedtime. The nighttime is the most efficient time to absorb calcium.

» Get sunshine as much as possible. Vitamin D is needed for your body to absorb calcium. Twenty minute of sunshine can supply enough vitamin D.

» Eat calcium-rich food such as lean meat, milk, eggs, oysters, soybeans, and seafood. Eat more celery, kelp, Chinese chive, tofu, bok choy, red dates, olives, bananas, and nuts. Add a little rice vinegar to your diet to help the absorption of calcium. Or you can take 1 tsp. of apple cider vinegar before each meal. Eat boron-rich foods such as apples, pears, grapes, or nuts. Boron is especially important for elderly women. Eat manganese-rich food such as milk, meat, and eggs.

» Exercising regularly is very important to build strong bones. Tai Chi, walking, and dancing are the best choices.

» If you have osteoporosis, be aware some medication will affect calcium absorption. Please consult with your doctor.

WHAT SHOULDN'T YOU DO?

» Don't eat too much sugar or salty food. Don't drink too much coffee or carbonated drinks. Sugar, salt, and caffeine will cause your body to lose calcium.

» Avoid bending your body or kicking your legs. If you bend your back forward, don't stretch up suddenly.

» Don't smoke. If you drink, drink no more than 5 oz. of wine, or 1 oz. 80-proof liquor a day.

» Don't try to lose weight without consulting professionals. Many young women take to an unbalanced diet to control weight and enhance the risk for osteoporosis.

Food Therapy

☞ Eat pig's neck bone with kelp:

Ingredients: 2 lb. pig's neck bone, 4 oz. kelp (seaweed).

Procedure: Soak the kelp in water overnight. Shred the kelp and place with the bones in a pot with 6 cups of water. Bring to a boil. Reduce heat and simmer until they are very soft. Add condiments and eat once a week.

☞ Drink milk with sesame powder:

Ingredients: 200 ml milk, 1/2 oz. sesame seed powder, honey.

Procedure: Mix with 1 tsp. of honey. Drink three times a day.

☞ Eat rice soup with herb:

Ingredients: 3 oz. rice, 1 oz. soybean powder, 1/2 oz. walnuts, 1/2 oz. black sesame seeds, 5 red dates, 1/4 oz. astragalus root, 1/2 oz. Chinese yam.

Procedure: Add 4 cups of water to all ingredients. Bring to a boil. Reduce heat and simmer for 20 minutes. Discard the astragalus. Eat frequently.

Chinese Massage

Massage the following points once a day:

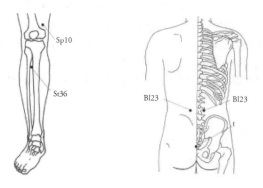

☞ Lie down on your stomach. Ask a family member to do the following:

　☞ Use the palm to gently rub your back two finger-widths either side of the spine, from the big neck bone down to the waist. Repeat two or three times.

☞ Use the palm to gently rub and knead your spine from the upper back down to the tip of tailbone. Repeat two or three times.

☞ Use the palm to knead the point at the base of the tailbone until it feels warm (Gv2).

☞ Use the tip of the middle finger to knead the points a little higher than the waist, two finger-widths on both sides of the spine for one minute (Bl23).

☞ Use the index finger to knead the point on the top of inside edge of the knee for one minute each side. Flex your knee and place your hand on the kneecap. The point is where your thumb touches (Sp10).

☞ Use the index finger to gently press the depression four finger-widths below the kneecap edge and one thumb's-width outside of the shinbone for one minute (St36).

Chinese Herbs

☞ If you have cold limbs, an aversion to cold, and general lassitude, take the patent herb Shen Qi Wan. Follow the instructions.

☞ If you have night sweats, irritability, thirst, blurred eyes, and tiredness, take the patent herb Liu Wei Di Huang Wan. Follow the instructions.

☞ If you have a weak digestive system, take the patent herb Xiang Sha Liu Jun Zi Wan to improve the ability for absorbing calcium and Vitamin D. Follow the instructions.

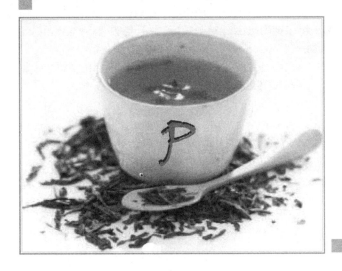

Peptic Ulcers

WHAT IS IT AND WHAT CAUSES IT?

Peptic ulcers are lesions in the inner lining of the stomach or duodenum. Some people can be symptom free. You may have pain in the upper abdomen or under the breastbone, a poor appetite, nausea, or bloating. If you have internal bleeding, you may have bloody or black, tar-like stool. It comes and goes. If the pain happens after a meal it is a *gastric ulcer*. If the pain appears two or four hours after a meal, it is a *duodenal ulcer*. Research shows the bacteria, called *helicobacter pylori,* is the main cause of peptic ulcers. Also genetics, some medications, a diet with too much fatty or spicy foods, smoking, or emotional stress can be other possible causes.

WHEN SHOULD YOU SEE A DOCTOR?

If you have any symptoms of peptic ulcers, see a doctor. If you are vomiting blood or have bloody or tar-like stool you need immediate medical attention.

WHAT SHOULD YOU DO IN DAILY LIFE?

* Take care of your ulcer in the early stages. As long as you have these symptoms and your breath has an unusually foul odor, see your doctor. It will be much easier to treat.

* Always eat on schedule. Eat small meals and do so more frequently. Eat easily digested food only.

* Drink more water. Eat yogurt instead of drinking milk. Eat ripe bananas and honey frequently. All this can protect the affected area in your stomach. Chewing gum produces more saliva, which could neutralize acid.

* Controlling your emotions is very important in your recovery process. Any upset, such as anger, fear, or depression, can disturb your internal secretion and accelerate the ulcer-forming process.

* Take it easy. Overexertion is another trigger for ulcers. Set up a reasonable work and rest schedule and follow it strictly. Sleep on time. Get out of bed on time.

* Watch medication such as painkillers. If you are taking aspirin or ibuprofen, ask your doctor to change your treatment.

WHAT SHOULDN'T YOU DO?

* Quitting smoking and drinking alcohol are very important steps for an ulcer patient.

* Don't eat too much. A large quantity of food will produce too much workload on the stomach and cause an ulcer.

* Absolutely avoid raw, cold foods and fried or greasy foods. Do not eat food that is hard to digest.

* Don't eat foods that are too sweet, too sour, too salty, or too hot. Drink less coffee and less strong tea. Don't drink soda.

Folk Remedies

☞ Use your four fingers to pat the back of opposite hand, the reflex zone of your stomach, for three minutes. Change hands and do the same. Continue for a prolonged period.

☞ Take potato charcoal:

Ingredients: 4 lb. potatoes.

Procedure: Crush potatoes in a blender until it looks like thick soup. Pour it into a cotton-fabric sack. Place the sack into 3 cups of clear water. Continuously squeeze or knead until a white paste-like powder appears. Pour this liquid into a pot and boil until almost dry. Lower the heat and bake it until brown. When it looks like a black film, grind the film to fine powder and store in a bottle. Take 1/4 tsp. before meals, three times a day for three weeks.

Food Therapy

☞ Take honey: Steam 100 ml honey in a bowl. Divide into three portions. Take one portion on an empty stomach three times a day for three weeks.

☞ Drink egg soup:

Ingredients: 1 egg.

Procedure: Beat the egg and boil in water. Eat 30 minutes before breakfast and bedtime every day.

☞ Eat sesame seeds with brown sugar and honey:

Ingredients: Sesame seeds, brown sugar, honey.

Procedure: Stir-fry sesame seeds until well done. In the same proportion mix the sesame, brown sugar, and honey together. Store in a bottle. Take 1 Tbs. before bedtime.

☞ Take ginger rice soup:

Ingredients: 1/8 oz. ginger, 3 oz. rice.

Procedure: Smash ginger to small pieces. Simmer ginger with 4 cups of water until only 3 cups are left. Strain out the residue. Add cooked rice to make rice soup. Drink once a day.

☞ Eat sticky rice with red dates:

Ingredients: 3 oz. sticky rice, 7 red dates, 25 ml honey.

Procedure: Add ingredients to 3 cups of water. Cook for 20 minutes to make a very soft rice soup. Drink twice a day for a week.

Chinese Massage

Choose the following points and massage once a day. If you have bloody stool, don't do massage.

☞ Gently push from the point halfway between the belly button (navel) and the low end of the breastbone (Cv12) to the lower end of your breastbone for two minutes. Gently press and knead Cv12 point for one minute.

☞ Gently rub the upper abdomen clockwise 100 times and counterclockwise 100 times. Don't press too hard.

☞ Gently press and knead the point two thumb-widths on cither side of the belly button for one minute (St25).

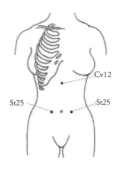 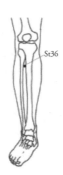 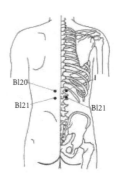

- Gently press the depression four finger-widths below the kneecap edge and one thumb's-width outside of the shinbone (St36).
- Gently press and knead the points on your back two finger widths apart from the spine on both sides, from four finger-widths above the waist all the way down to the waistline for one minute (Bl20, Bl21).

Chinese Herbs

- If you have a dull stomach pain that feels better with warmth, pressure, or after a meal, take the patent herb Fu Zi Li Zhong Wan. Follow the instructions.
- If you have stomach pain radiating to your ribs related to emotional upset, a sensation of bloating, belching, a sensation of bitterness, or acid reflux, take the patent herb Chai Hu Shu Gan Wan. Follow the instructions.
- If you have stomach pain with a burning sensation that radiates to the ribs and is not alleviated by eating a meal, and you are feeling irritable and have bitter sensations in your mouth, take the patent herb Zuo Jin Wan. Follow the instructions.
- If you have stitching stomach pain at a fixed area that is worse with pressure, or black stool, take lotus and egg with herbs:

    Ingredients: 1/8 oz. pseudoginseng powder, 3 oz. lotus root, 1 egg.

    Procedure: Use a juicer to make lotus juice first. Beat an egg. Place the egg, lotus juice, and herbs in a bowl. Steam them for 20 minutes. Eat twice a day.

Prostate Problems

WHAT IS IT AND WHAT CAUSES IT?

Enlargement of the prostate and prostatitis are conditions common in men older than age 40. Enlargement of the prostate is called benign prostatic hyperplasia (BPH). Symptoms are frequent urination at night, delayed urination, a weak urine stream, and dribbling. The cause of BPH still remains unclear. It may be related to hormones. Prostatitis is an inflammation of the prostate gland caused by urine trapped in the bladder. Symptoms are burning, painful, and frequent urination, pain in the perineum area and lower back, impotence, and fever.

WHEN SHOULD YOU SEE A DOCTOR?

If you are experiencing any urination problems, see your doctor.

WHAT SHOULD YOU DO IN DAILY LIFE?

* Stress, depression, or anxiety can contribute to a prostate problem. You should keep an optimistic outlook. Keep yourself upbeat by chatting, walking, dancing, or listening to music. Understanding the cure of a prostate problem is a long-term process. Increasing your confidence, and persistently getting treatments are the key factors for recovering.
* Eat more vegetables and fruits. Eat zinc-rich food such as sesame seeds, watermelon, pumpkin seeds, oyster, fish, apples, and apricots. Eat two or three tomatoes a day.
* Drink plenty of water to encourage urination before noon.
* Sleep with a hot water bottle. The temperature should be as hot as is comfortable. Place the bottle on the lower abdomen just below the bellybutton. It will help to decrease frequent urination at night.
* Take a warm bath for 20 minutes before bedtime. Meanwhile, use a warm towel to massage the area between the anus and testicles.

» Exercise regularly. Jogging and practicing Tai Chi are good for recovering from prostate illnesses. This kind of exercise can act as an internal massage to the prostate.

WHAT SHOULDN'T YOU DO?

» Avoid spicy and greasy foods. Drink less soda, coffee, and tea. Eat less acidic foods such as citrus fruits and orange juice. Avoid hot-natured foods such as ginger, garlic, or cinnamon.

» Don't ride a bicycle or sit for a prolonged period of time. Never sit on damp or cold ground.

» Quit smoking. Drink less alcohol.

» Avoid constipation.

Folk Remedies

☞ Sound therapy for difficult urination: Place a container under a water tap. Open the tap slightly and let water drip into the container. Record the sound of the drops and play the tape when you want to urinate.

☞ Vision therapy for difficult urination: Hang a picture or painting with a waterfall flowing down from a mountain on the wall behind the toilet.

☞ For frequent urination at night, use your palms to gently tap both sides of the back at the level of the waist 150 to 200 times rhythmically.

☞ To treat enlargement of prostate, apply salt to your lower abdomen. Stir-fry salt and place in a cotton bag. Apply to the midline of your lower abdomen for 30 minutes. Take care not to burn yourself. Reheat the salt if it becomes cool.

☞ For prostatitis, drink royal bee jelly. It is available in Chinese grocery stores. Dilute the jelly with water to make 1 to 100 solution (for example, mix one Tbs. of royal bee jelly with 6 cups of water). Drink 30 ml at a time on an empty stomach, three times a day for a prolonged period.

Food Therapy

- For prostatitis, drink sugarcane juice. Peel 1 lb. of sugarcane. Use a juicer to make juice. Divide into two portions and drink twice a day.
- Eat six cloves of slightly fried, warm walnuts before bedtime every day.
- To treat enlargement of prostate, take raw pumpkins seeds (1 oz. a day). Or take pumpkin powder (2 or 3 tsp. a day).
- For prostatitis drink Chinese cabbage and lotus tea:

    Ingredients: 1 lb. Chinese cabbage root, 1 lb. lotus root.

    Procedure: Slice the cabbage root into small pieces. Remove the node of lotus and slice into small pieces. Use a juicer to make juice separately. Mix these juices and drink before bedtime.

Chinese Massage

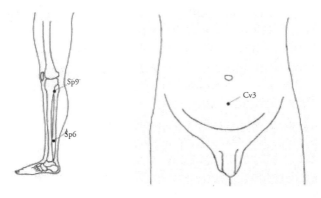

- If you have difficulty urinating, use your thumb to gently press the point right at the midpoint between the pubic bone and belly button (navel). Start with mild pressure and gradually increase the force until all urine passes.
- As routine exercise, choose from the following and massage once a day for a prolonged period:

- Lie down on a bed. Rub your palms together until they feel warm. Place your left palm on your belly button. Overlap your right palm. Gently rub the lower abdomen clockwise for two minutes, then rub counterclockwise for another two minutes. Place both palms on either side of the belly button and push down to the top of the legs for two minutes.

- Use your fingers to rub and knead your lower back down to the sacral area for two minutes. Use your palm to gently pat that area for one minute.

- Sit on a chair or lie down on a bed. Use your right middle finger to gently knead the perineum, the area between the anus and scrotum, for two minutes.

- Use the middle finger to gently press the point on the midline of the lower abdomen about one hand's-width below the belly button (Cv3). Gradually press down a little deeper, and press toward the perineum until you have a sensation of distention. Continue the pressure for 30 seconds then quickly release. Repeat three times.

- Gently press and knead the point right in the depression inside of the calf under the knee, behind the leg bone (Sp9), and the point four finger-widths up from the inside anklebone, right behind the leg bone (Sp6).

Qi Gong

- Stand with your feet shoulder width apart in a quiet room. Relax, and breathe naturally.

- While inhaling, squeeze the sphincter muscles around the anus, perineum, and tailbone. (Similar to holding a bowel movement.)

- While exhaling, slowly loosen the sphincter muscles around the anus, perineum, and tailbone. (Similar to the feeling when you are urinating.)

- Repeat for two minutes, twice a day for three weeks.

Chinese Herbs

- To treat prostatitis, insert the patent herb wild chrysanthemum suppository into your anus, twice a day for two weeks. Consult your doctor before using this product.
- For enlargement of prostate, take American ginseng and pseudoginseng:

   Ingredients: 1/2 oz. pseudoginseng, 1/2 oz. American ginseng.

   Procedure: Grind each herb into fine powder. Mix well. Take 1/8 oz. at a time with warm water, once a day. One course is 15 days. Repeat for two or three courses.

Psoriasis

WHAT IS IT AND WHAT CAUSES IT?

Psoriasis is a skin disease with red, itchy, raised patches covered by white scales that can fall in flakes. The cause of psoriasis still remains unclear. It may be related to stress, alcohol, and weather, or it can be genetic.

WHEN SHOULD YOU SEE A DOCTOR?

If you suspect your skin problem is psoriasis, see a doctor. If the psoriatic patches spread wildly, or if you have fever or joint pain, visit your doctor immediately.

WHAT SHOULD YOU DO IN DAILY LIFE?

- Relax, as excessive stress is one of the triggers. Maintain a positive attitude about your life and current situation. Don't take things too hard. Listening to soft music 15 minutes in the sunshine is a good way to reduce stress.
- Before applying any medications, use warm water and mild soap to wash the infected area carefully. Scrape off the flakes or scales.

- Sunbathing in bright and warm weather is very helpful. Begin with 10 minutes and gradually extend to one hour. Wear sunglasses to protect your eyes. Take a mineral bath if possible.
- Take enough vitamins. Eat more omega-3 rich food such as salmon.
- Exercise such as walking and Tai Chi should be done regularly.

WHAT SHOULDN'T YOU DO?

- Don't scratch. Instead, pat the affected spot to suppress itching. Applying a towel soaked in cold milk may provide relief from itching.
- Avoid spicy, greasy foods. Don't eat lamb, fish, shrimp, chives, onion, garlic, cinnamon, hot pepper, mustard, or fennel fruit, which will stimulate psoriasis.
- No alcohol at all.
- Don't stop using current medication without consulting your doctor first.
- If your psoriasis is in a developing stage, avoid any damage or stimulation to your normal skin such as injection, or any injury, which will cause new flare-ups.

Folk Remedies

- Wash infected spot as much as possible. Take a warm bath frequently with 1/2 cup of ground oatmeal. Use only very gentle, mild soap with additional moisturizers. Apply a thick layer of heavy cream to keep your skin moist.
- Use banana peels (inner side) to rub the infected area for a prolonged period. Applying aloe vera gel will help too. If you have an allergic reaction, discontinue use.
- Use a low-power vacuum cleaner to alleviate your itching. Remove the head or brush of the vacuum cleaner. Use the opening of the pipe to gently suck at your bellybutton (navel). Try to slightly lift the pipe, but don't lose contact with the skin. Continue for 10 seconds with suction. Repeat several times.

☞ Wash with willow branch water:

Ingredients: Fresh willow branches.

Procedure: Cut the willow branch into 3-inch stems. Put them in a pot with adequate water. Bring to a boil. Lower the heat to simmer until water becomes black. Wash the infected spot three times a day. The use of elm tree is also good. If you have an allergic reaction, stop.

☞ Apply water chestnuts and vinegar:

Ingredients: 15 water chestnuts, 90 ml rice vinegar.

Procedure: Slice water chestnuts and soak in vinegar. Simmer for 10 minutes. After the water chestnuts absorb the vinegar, crush the chestnuts and store in a sealed jar. Apply to the infected area, and cover with a piece of gauze. Change it daily. If you have an allergic reaction, discontinue use.

Food Therapy

☞ Eat Chinese dried mushrooms for a prolonged period. Soak in water for two hours. Stir-fry with cooking oil and soybean sauce. Eat with other foods.

☞ Eat black plums.

Ingredients: 1 lb. black plum, sugar.

Procedure: Remove the center. Add 2 cups of water and bring to a boil. Reduce heat and simmer until it becomes very thick. Store in a sealed jar. Take 1 Tbs. at a time with 1 tsp. of sugar, three times a day.

Chinese Massage

Gently press and knead the following points for one or two minutes:

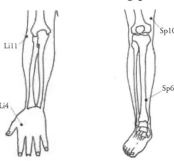

- When your thumb is against the index finger, the webbing where it bulges up the highest (Li4).
- The point at the end of the crease on the top of the elbow joint, when the arm is folded across the chest for one minute (Li11).
- The point four finger-widths up from the inside anklebone, right behind the leg bone (Sp6).
- The point on the top of inside edge of the knee. Flex your knee and place your hand on the kneecap. The point is where your thumb touches (Sp10).

Chinese Herbs

- Take the patent herb Wu Shao She Pia. Follow the instructions.

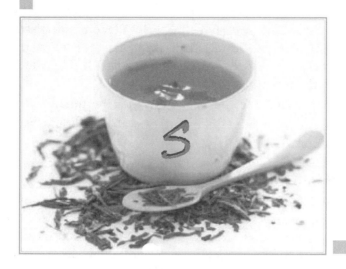

Sciatica

WHAT IS IT AND WHAT CAUSES IT?

Sciatica is a pain along the sciatic nerve and its branches. The nerve originates in the back, and continues through the hip and down the leg. The pain is dull or sharp, is mostly on one side, and gets worse at night. Nerve root inflammation or the compression of a nerve root in the back are the main causes of sciatica.

WHEN SHOULD YOU SEE A DOCTOR?

See a doctor if you have severe pain, or after self-treatment for three days you have no success, or you have numbness in your leg and foot.

WHAT SHOULD YOU DO IN DAILY LIFE?

* Sleep on a hard mattress.
* For acute cases use a cold compress. Apply a cold gel pack or small plastic bag with ice wrapped with a cloth to the painful spot for 20 minutes three times a day. After one or two days, apply a heating pad for 20 minutes several times a day.

255

* Use chairs with firm support and sit back in your chair to avoid concentrated pressure on the sciatic nerve. If you work at a desk for prolonged time, adjust the height of your desk and chair properly. Place a small stool or box under your desk. Place your feet on it to raise your knee joint higher than the pelvic joint. In this way, your sciatic nerve has less pressure.
* Keep your back and limbs warm all the time.
* Exercises such as swimming or walking should be done regularly.

WHAT SHOULDN'T YOU DO?

* Avoid walking in the rain. If you are sweating, don't expose yourself to the wind. Change your underwear as soon as possible if you get wet. Never sleep directly on the ground or sit on a rock or a wet chair. Dampness and cold are the factors that can cause sciatica.
* Avoid crossing your legs when you are sitting.

Folk Remedies

* Apply tofu with vinegar:

    Ingredients: Tofu, rice vinegar.

    Procedure: Cut a 1/4-inch slice of tofu and use a fork to punch a lot of holes in it. In acute cases, freeze the tofu in a refrigerator for three minutes. Soak it in a bowl with vinegar. Apply to the painful area for 15 minutes. In chronic cases, use a microwave to warm the tofu and apply to the painful area for 20 minutes. Reheat the tofu if necessary. If you have an allergic skin reaction, stop.

* In chronic cases, remove the head or brush of a low-power vacuum cleaner. Use the opening of the pipe to gently suck your back muscles. Try to slightly lift the pipe, but don't lose contact with the skin. Continue for 10 seconds with suction at each spot while moving the pipe along the painful area down your leg.

☙ If your pain is worse with cold, apply green onion paste:

Ingredients: 6 pieces of white stalk of green onion.

Procedure: Slice into small pieces. Stir-fry until warm, then wrap with a piece of cotton. Apply to the painful area for 20 minutes. If you have an allergic reaction, discontinue use.

Food Therapy

☙ Drink vegetable juice:

Ingredients: 10 oz. carrots, 10 oz. potato, 7 oz. celery, 7 oz. apple, 30 ml honey.

Procedure: Use a juicer to make juice of potato, celery, carrot, and apple. Add honey. Drink daily.

☙ Drink herb wine:

Ingredients: 1 oz. salvia, 500 ml 80-proof vodka.

Procedure: Cut salvia into small pieces. Soak in vodka in a sealed bottle for 15 days. Shake every day. Drink 20 ml with 30 ml water, twice a day.

☙ If the painful area is feeling warm, becoming worse in hot weather or on wet days, make the following soup:

Ingredients: 2 oz. Chinese pearl barley, 2 oz. mung beans.

Procedure: Soak beans in water overnight. Add 4 cups of water and cook on low heat until beans are soft. Divide into two portions, and drink twice a day for a week.

☙ If your pain becomes worse with cold and alleviated with heat, but is not better with rest, make the following soup:

Ingredients: 1/8 oz. dried ginger, 1/4 oz. poria, 5 red dates, 3 oz. rice, 1 Tbs. brown sugar.

Procedure: Wrap dried ginger with gauze. Place herbs into a pot. Add 2 cups of water. Bring to a boil, reduce heat and simmer for 20 minutes. Add rice, dates, sugar, and 2 cups of water. Continue to cook on low heat for 20 minutes. Discard dried ginger. Divide into two portions and eat twice a day for three days.

❧ If you have stitching painthat is fixed in one region and tender to touch, and is worse at night, drink the following wine:

Ingredients: 1 oz. safflower, 1 oz. salvia, 1 oz. millettia stem, 2,000 ml Chinese cooking wine.

Procedure: Soak herbs in wine for three days. Drink 20 ml at a time, twice a day.

❧ If you experience dull pain that is worse with exertion, and weakness in the back and knee, make the following rice soup:

Ingredients: 2 oz. Chinese yam, 1 oz. lycium fruit, 3 oz. rice.

Procedure: Wrap lycium with gauze. Add 2 cups of water. Bring to a boil. Reduce heat and simmer for 20 minutes. Strain the liquid into a pot. Add rice and 2 cups of water. Continue to cook for 20 minutes. Eat once a day for a week.

Chinese Massage

Choose the following and massage each for one or two minutes once a day. In an acute case, don't massage the painful spots.

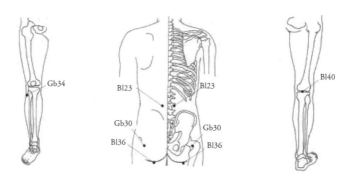

❧ Sit on a chair and with loose fists, gently and continuously pat your lower back and sacral bone area.

❧ Locate the most painful spot. Using your thumb, flick that spot several times, then gently press and knead.

- Use both palms to push the muscles from the thigh down to the lower leg.
- Press and knead the point a little higher than the waist, two finger-widths on both sides of the spine (Bl23).
- Press the points on the side of your buttocks. You can find this point by placing your thumbs on your hipbones, opening all fingers, and resting your little fingers around the back. The ends of your middle fingers are at the points (Gb30).
- Press the center of the fold where the leg and buttocks meet on both sides (Bl36).
- Sit on a chair and use your thumb to gently press the point outside of the leg, under the kneecap edge in the depression below the two lower leg bones' meeting point (Gb34).
- Use the thumb to gently press the point in the middle of the crease on the back of the knee (Bl40).

Chinese Herbs

- Take the patent herbs Mu Gua Wan, Du Huo Ji Sheng Wan, or Vine Essence Pill. Follow the instructions.
- Apply a heating patch with herb, called Chinese Moxibustion. Follow the instructions.

Sexual Desire (Lowered)

WHAT IS IT AND WHAT CAUSES IT?

Hypoactive sexual desire is not only related to aging. It could also be related to a physical illness, medication, stress, or psychological factors. Sometimes the pain from intercourse or unreasonable expectations may contribute to the loss of interest for sex. Symptoms include diminished sexual desire and a lack of sexual fantasies.

WHEN SHOULD YOU SEE A DOCTOR?

If your sexual desires are low and have been for a long period of time and it affects your relationship with your partner, or if you feel no improvement after self-treatment, see a doctor.

WHAT SHOULD YOU DO IN DAILY LIFE?

- ✻ The frequency of sex should follow the rule of nature. You should have sex only when your mental and physical conditions are in good shape. If you find less drive, consider sleeping temporarily in another room. Give your nervous system and endocrine system some time to adjust to a normal level.

- ✻ Eat more shrimp, lamb, beef, Chinese chive, carrots, turtle, and walnuts. In Chinese medicine, they strengthen the sexual organs.

- ✻ Taking a hot bath before intimate activities can improve blood circulation in your sex organs.

- ✻ Be aware that some medications may make you have less of a drive for sex.

- ✻ If you have constipation, treat promptly. In many cases, constipation may cause you to lose sexual desires.

WHAT SHOULDN'T YOU DO?

- ✻ Don't think of sex as a job you have to do. Think of it as a natural highlight of your mutual feelings. Any romantic gestures, kissing, and gentle caresses will play an important role in making you and your partner more desirable to each other.

- ✻ No alcohol. For women drinking moderately can increase the sexual desire. But if you become alcoholic, it makes your desire worse. Drink less coffee and strong tea.

Food Therapy

- ☞ Take rice soup with lycium:

    Ingredients: 2 oz. rice. 1 oz. lycium fruit.

    Procedure: Add 3 cups of water to rice and cook for 20 minutes to make rice soup. During the last five minutes, add lycium fruit. Drink the soup as you like.

- ☞ Drink royal jelly:

    Ingredients: 60 ml royal jelly, 60 ml honey.

    Procedure: Mix them well. Take 15 ml at a time, once or twice a day.

☞ Eat shrimp with Chinese chive:

Ingredients: 8 oz. shrimp, 8 oz. Chinese chive, cooking oil, salt.

Procedure: Stir-fry shrimp in oil until well done. Slice chives into 1-inch strips. Stir-fry chives with oil. Add salt and mix with shrimp. Eat this once a week.

☞ Eat gecko with pilose deer horn:

Ingredients: A pair of geckos, 3/4 oz. sliced pilose deer horn, Chinese cooking wine. The ingredients are available in Chinese herb stores.

Procedure: Soak the gecko in clear water overnight. Cut off the head and legs and remove the black skin. Place them on a piece of aluminum foil to dry with low heat. Lightly bake deer horn. Grind both to fine powder. Take 1/8 oz. with Chinese cooking wine before bedtime. If you feel irritable or uncomfortable, stop.

Chinese Herbs

☞ If you feel it is caused by deficiency (feel too tired to have sex), for a woman, take the patent herb Wu Ji Bai Feng Wan; for a man, take the patent herb Nan Bao. Follow the instructions.

☞ If you feel it is caused by stress, for women, take the patent herb Dan Zhi Xiao Yao Wan; for men, take the patent herb Xiao Yao Wan. Follow the instructions.

Shin Splints

WHAT IS IT AND WHAT CAUSES IT?

Shin splints refer to a "splintering" pain of the shinbone area, accompanied by swelling of the tissue. It arises from excessive stress, which can be caused by over exercising.

WHEN SHOULD YOU SEE A DOCTOR?

If the symptoms persist, you need to see a doctor to make sure you don't have a more serious condition, such as a stress fracture.

WHAT SHOULD YOU DO IN DAILY LIFE?

- ✈ Wear shoes that offer good arch support.
- ✈ Stretch or massage your leg before and after exercising.
- ✈ Alternately apply a heat pack and ice pack to the shin every 10 to 20 minutes.
- ✈ Change shoes daily.

WHAT SHOULDN'T YOU DO?

- ✈ Don't participate in strenuous activities.

Folk Remedies

- ☙ Freeze a block of tofu for two minutes. Use a fork to puncture a lot of holes in the tofu. Cut a 1/4-inch slice. Soak this slice in rice vinegar for three seconds. Apply it to the painful area for 15 minutes. If you have an allergic reaction, stop.

Chinese Massage

Stand up, and lift the afflicted leg on a chair:

- ☙ Use both hands to gently slap up and down the sides of the leg 20 times.
- ☙ Use the heel of both palms to gently push the muscles from your knee down to the ankle 20 times.
- ☙ Use your thumb and other four fingers to grasp the muscles from the knee down to the ankle 20 times.

Chinese Herbs

- ☙ Take the patent herb Yun Nan Bai Yao. Follow the instructions.

Shingles (Herpes Zoster)

WHAT IS IT AND WHAT CAUSES IT?

Shingles is a disease caused by the virus called varicella zoster. The symptoms are severe pain and itching, with a band-like red rash of fluid-filled blisters. It is caused by a reactivated chicken pox virus inside nerve tissue.

WHEN SHOULD YOU SEE A DOCTOR?

If you start to have a skin condition like the previously mentioned one, see a doctor. If you have shingles affecting your nose and eyes, see a doctor immediately.

WHAT SHOULD YOU DO IN DAILY LIFE?

- Eat more watermelon, cucumber, radish, winter melon, bitter melon, pineapple, mung beans, or green beans.
- Take it easy. Emotional upset is one of the triggers.
- Have regular bowel movements. Avoid constipation.
- Wear cotton, soft clothes. If a blister is broken, change your underwear. Wash your hands frequently.

WHAT SHOULDN'T YOU DO?

- Don't try to break the blister. If the blister is broken, wash it right away.
- Don't use hot water to suppress the itching. Instead apply a towel soaked in cold milk to the affected area.
- Don't eat fried food and spicy foods such as ginger, garlic, chili pepper, or fennel. Avoid over stimulating foods such as lamb, shrimp, or crab.
- No alcohol.

Folk Remedies

When you use the following remedies, if you have an allergic reaction, discontinue use:

- Spread baking soda over the infected area. You can also mix it with water to make paste and apply it.
- Apply aloe vera juice or 100-percent aloe vera gel.
- Apply fig leaves. Wash and pound fig leaves. Mix with rice vinegar to make paste and apply to the affected area.
- Apply cactus paste:
    Ingredients: Fresh cactus, sticky rice powder.

Procedure: Remove the needles and pound it well. Mix with a little sticky rice powder to make paste. Apply to lesions and change it if it becomes dry.

Food Therapy

☞ If you have a red rash on the chest with pain like fire, a sensation of bitterness in the mouth, poor appetite, and you feel fidgety, drink rice soup with herbs:

Ingredients: 1/8 oz. isatis leaf, 1/8 oz. bupleurum, 1 oz. rice, sugar.

Procedure: Put isatis leaf and bupleurum in a pot. Add 3 cups of water. Bring to a boil. Reduce heat and simmer until 2/3 of the water remains. Strain and add rice and sugar. Continue to cook for 20 minutes to make rice soup. Drink once a day for five days.

☞ If you have a light-red rash on the lower limbs or clusters of pus-filled blisters on the abdomen, loose stools, and you feel bloated after meals, you can eat the following soup:

Ingredients: 1 oz. Chinese pearl barley, 1 oz. purslane, brown sugar.

Procedure: Add 3 cups of water to the barley and purslane. Bring to a boil. Reduce heat and simmer for 20 minutes. Add 1 tsp. sugar and eat once a day for five days.

☞ If you have a few blisters, or blisters that burst and crust over with pale scars that are painful, drink egg soup with herbs:

Ingredients: 1/8 oz. bupleurum, 1/8 oz. dang gui, 1/8 oz. tangerine peels, 1 egg.

Procedure: Place herbs in a pot. Add 2 cups of water and bring to a boil. Reduce heat and simmer for 20 minutes. Strain the decoction and discard herb residue. Beat an egg. Bring the decoction to a boil again. Pour the egg and stir well. Eat the egg and drink the decoction, once a day for five days.

Chinese Massage

Using your thumb, gently press and knead any combination of the following points for one minute to relieve your pain:

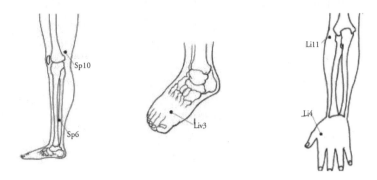

- The point on the inside edge of the top of the knee. Flex your knee and place your hand on the kneecap. The point is where your thumb touches (Sp10).
- The point at the end of the crease on the top of the elbow joint, when the arm is folded across the chest (Li11).
- With your thumb against the index finger, the webbing where it bulges up the highest (Li4).
- The point four finger-widths up from the inside ankle-bone, right behind the leg bone (Sp6).
- The point between the big and second toes, two finger-widths up the foot from the joint between the toes (Liv3).

Chinese Herbs

- Apply the patent herb Liu Shen Wan. Depending on the size of the infected area, grind 100 or 200 pills of Liu Shen Wan into a fine powder. Apply it directly to the affected spot, if blisters are already broken. Otherwise mix the powder with rice vinegar and apply. If you have an allergic reaction, discontinue use.

Shoulder Pain (Chronic)

WHAT IS IT AND WHAT CAUSES IT?

Shoulder pain may have many causes. There are three common types:

* Frozen shoulder. Severe pain in the shoulder with restricted motion. It is caused by an inflammation in the shoulder joint.
* Rotator cuff injury. It is the tear, strain, or rupture of the muscles or tendons that link the upper arm and shoulder blade. It is often caused by too much overhead arm activities, or simply by aging.
* Osteoarthritis is another possible cause of shoulder pain.

WHEN SHOULD YOU SEE A DOCTOR?

If you can't move your arm, your pain is severe, or your pain does not respond to self-treatment, see a doctor.

WHAT SHOULD YOU DO IN DAILY LIFE?

* Select the correct pillow to keep your spine in a natural position when sleeping. This could prevent a sore shoulder, especially for the elderly.
* Always keep your shoulder warm. Never sleep outside or let your shoulder face an open window. In hot weather don't expose your shoulder to an electric fan for a long period of time.
* Move and exercise your shoulder. Do it gradually. Don't expect the pain to go away in a very short time. Passive movement might be a good first step. If you ask somebody to help to do passive movement, begin very slowly and gently. Exercise is crucial for recovering your shoulder function.
* For an acute case, apply ice on the painful spot for 15 to 20 minutes, three times a day. When the inflammation is gone, apply a heating pad for 20 minutes three times a day.
* Eat more warm and tonifying food such as lamb, walnuts, ginger, and Chinese chive. Eat more tofu and other bean products.

- In chronic cases, take a hot bath (as hot as you feel comfortable) regularly. If you can't raise or move your arm, you should do following exercises during your bath or right after:
  - Put your palm on the wall and move your fingers up slowly to bring arm towards the ceiling. Slowly raise your arm as high as you can. When you reach your limit, stay there for 10 seconds. Then slowly move downwards.
  - Slowly bend your painful arm backwards, trying to reach your upper back. Gradually move to the point you can reach forward.
  - Slowly raise and bend your elbow. Try to reach the top of your ear on the same side. Then try to cross your arm over your head and reach the top of your ear on the other side.
  - After you are dressed, standing in the middle of the room, slowly rotate your arm forward or backward like swimming freestyle or doing the backstroke for two minutes.

WHAT SHOULDN'T YOU DO?

- Don't wear high heel shoes. This may be the cause of your shoulder pain.
- Avoid cold food.

Folk Remedies

- When you are bathing, use a hairbrush to lightly tap your shoulder for five minutes. This will stimulate your body like many acupuncture needles. Begin at the base of your neck out to the side of each shoulder, then from the neck downwards to the upper back. If it is acute don't do this.
- In chronic cases use a low power vacuum cleaner to massage your shoulder. Remove the head or brush of the vacuum cleaner. Use the opening of the pipe to gently suck at the following points. Try to slightly lift the pipe, but don't lose contact with the skin. Continue for 10 seconds with suction. Repeat this procedure two times.

- ☙ The most painful spot.
- ☙ The points under the earlobes, right at the top of the shoulders (Gb21).
- ☙ The point on the top of the shoulder in the front depression formed when your arm is raised parallel to the ground (Li15).

☙ In a chronic case apply potato hot paste:

Ingredients: 1 potato, 1 Tbs. flour.

Procedure: Make potato paste with a blender. Squeeze out the excess water. Mix the potato with flour. Place on a piece of gauze and apply to the painful spot on your shoulder. Cover with clear plastic wrap and a heating pad for 10 minutes. Repeat this procedure two times a day for one week.

☙ Apply tofu with vinegar:

Ingredients: tofu, rice vinegar.

Procedure: cut a quarter-inch slice of tofu and use a fork to punch a lot of holes in it. In acute cases, freeze the tofu in a refrigerator for three minutes. Soak it in a bowl with vinegar. Apply to the painful area for 15 minutes. In chronic cases, use a microwave to warm the tofu and apply to the painful area for 20 minutes. Reheat the tofu if necessary. If you have an allergic skin reaction, discontinue use.

☙ Blow the pain away: Set a hair dryer to low. In a chronic case, blow hot air on the painful spot and from the kneecap down the outside, halfway of the leg for three minutes. In an acute case, only blow on the leg. If it feels too warm, move the hair dryer further away. Take care not to burn yourself.

☙ Play Chinese health balls, available in Chinese herb stores, for 20 minutes. You can use one ball at a time, or simultaneously use two in one hand. There are six meridians that run through the hand. Some of them go through the shoulder.

Food Therapy

- ☞ Drink lemon juice every day. Lemon will neutralize the lactic acid, which causes shoulder pain.
- ☞ Drink herb wine:

    Ingredients: 1/4 oz. safflower, 1/4 oz. cyathula root, 1/4 oz. ligusticum, 500 ml 80-proof vodka.

    Procedure: Soak herbs in vodka for one week. Shake well every day. Drink 15 ml with 20 ml water on an empty stomach, twice a day.

Chinese Massage

Choose the following points and massage each for one or two minutes. In an acute case, don't massage the painful spot.

- ☞ Use your fingers to gently press and knead the outside of your arm from the fingers to the shoulder. Then from inside of the arm down to the palm.

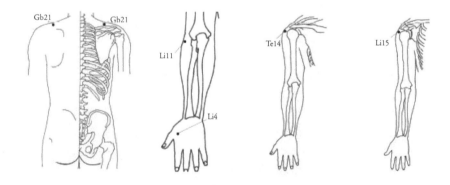

- ☞ Place your forearm on a table. Use your palm or fingers to rub, pat, and knead the painful area on your shoulder and upper arm, especially the front and outside. Start gently and gradually increase the pressure.
- ☞ Use the heel of your palm and four fingers to grasp the painful shoulder joint. Use your thumb, index, and middle fingers to grasp and pinch the tendon of your armpit.

- Swing your arms forward and backward for two minutes. Gradually increase the amplitude and the speed.

- Use your middle finger to gently press the points under the earlobes, right at the top of the shoulders (Gb21). Meanwhile, try to move your shoulder joint.

- Raise your arm parallel to the ground. Find a depression in front of the shoulder top (Li15). Use your middle finger to gently press this point. Slowly put your arm down and continue to press.

- Raise your arm sideways, parallel to the ground. Find a depression in back of the shoulder top (Te14). Use your middle finger to gently press this point. Slowly put your arm down and continue to press.

- Use your thumb to gently press the point at the end of the crease on the top of the elbow joint, when the arm is folded across the chest (Li11).

- With your thumb against the index finger, use your other thumb to gently press and knead the webbing where it bulges up the highest (Li4).

Chinese Herbs

- For an acute case, take the patent herb Mu Gua Wan. Follow the instructions.

- For a chronic case, take the patent herb Da Huo Luo Wan. Follow the instructions.

- Use the patent herb tincture Yu Nan Bai Yao to rub your shoulder. Follow the instructions.

- Apply a heating patch with herb, called Chinese Moxibustion. Follow the instructions.

Sinusitis

WHAT IS IT AND WHAT CAUSES IT?

Sinusitis is an inflammation and blockage of the sinus cavity caused by infection. Normally the sinuses humidify the air you breathe and trap harmful bacteria. When the air no longer flows freely, usually because of excess mucus produced during a cold, the bacteria start to grow and cause infection. The symptoms include fullness behind the face, facial pain, head congestion, fever, and headaches.

WHEN SHOULD YOU SEE A DOCTOR?

If the symptoms persist for more than a week, or you are running a high fever, see your doctor. If you feel pain or bulging in the eyes, nausea, or vomiting, see your doctor immediately.

WHAT SHOULD YOU DO IN DAILY LIFE?

* A hot shower can help drain the mucus and relieve the stiffness. Do it two times a day. Cup some water and pat it on your face around the nose area. Before and after the shower, drink plenty of water. Dehydration from sweating can make it worse.

* You may also use a facial steam machine that can blow warm steam into the nostrils. These machines are available in department stores.

* Keep your sinus cavity moist by using a humidifier in the room.

* Drink plenty of water. Drinking 8 cups of water a day will make the mucus thinner and relieve the blockage.

* Eat more coriander, oranges, tangerines, grapefruit, sweet apricot seeds, lily bulbs, or Chinese white fungus. These foods help to clear the nose.

* Exercise regularly by walking at least 30 minutes a day.

WHAT SHOULDN'T YOU DO?

* Do not blow your nose too violently. Instead, blow one nostril then the other, not together. The sudden pressure in your ears can push bacteria back to the sinuses.

- ❧ Don't eat spicy foods or consume tobacco and alcohol.
- ❧ Avoid polluted air. Avoid known allergens.
- ❧ Avoid bending your head down, as it increases pain.

Folk Remedies

- ☞ Use warm water to wash the nostrils and remove excess nasal discharge. For best results, use a saline solution in a medicine dropper or nasal spray.
- ☞ Use a dropper and drop two drops of sesame oil into your nostrils, twice a day.
- ☞ Chop 1 lb. of diakon radish into chunks and boil with water in a kettle. Wait until the vapors are not too hot. Open your mouth and breathe in the vapors. Don't scald yourself.
- ☞ Cover your ears with warm, wet towels for 10 minutes three times a day. If the sinuses clear up, repeat two times a day.
- ☞ Add 1/4 tsp. of table salt to 1 cup of water. Add 1 tsp. of green tea (best quality) and bring it to a boil. Wait until it cools to warm. Tip your head back, press one nostril closed, and use a dropper to pour some of the liquid into the other nostril. Lower your head and let the liquid flow out. Do three times in one nostril, then repeat with the other.

Chinese Massage

- ☞ Dry wash your face: Sit with your eyes closed. Rub your hands together until they are warm. Use your fingers to wipe your face from your forehead downward to the lips, to the lower jaw, to underneath the ears, then circle back upward to the temples. You should do this 10 times. Repeat in the opposite direction.
- ☞ Use your index, middle, and ring fingers together to gently knead clockwise the top of your head for one minute.
- ☞ Use both index fingers to tap the point in the middle of the groove, just outside the edge of the nostril for one minute (Li20).

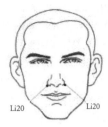

Li20   Li20

- Place your index finger at the lower left corner of your nose. Gently press and knead for 30 seconds. Then trace upward to the corner of the eye 30 times. Repeat this procedure on the other side.
- Rub the upper lip area and the spot on the cheek directly below your eyes.

Chinese Herbs

- If your mucus is thick green or yellowish, take the patent herb Bi Yan Pian. Follow the instructions.
- If your mucus is white or clear, take the patent herb Bi Min Gan Wan. Follow the instructions.

Sore Throat (Pharyngitis)

WHAT IS IT AND WHAT CAUSES IT?

Pharyngitis is an inflammation of the throat. Symptom is a raw, scratchy painful feeling in the throat with redness and swelling. It is caused by a viral or bacterial infection.

WHEN SHOULD YOU SEE A DOCTOR?

If you have a severe sore throat accompanied by a fever, or after two days it becomes worse, see a doctor. If it is difficult to swallow or breathe, go to an emergency room immediately.

WHAT SHOULD YOU DO IN DAILY LIFE?

- In an acute case, get plenty of rest. Limit using your voice too much.

- Keep your mouth clean. Use salt water (1 tsp. of salt with 2 cups of warm water) or diluted lemon juice to to gargle. Repeat five to 10 times a day, especially after meals.
- Drink a lot of water.
- Use your nose, not your mouth, to breathe. Wear a mask in an air-polluted place.
- Eat soft and easily digested food such as milk, rice soup, soybean milk, and oatmeal. Eat more fruits and vegetables such as Chinese cabbage, cucumber, tomatoes, lemons, olives, radishes, pears, and water chestnuts.
- Have regular bowel movements.
- If you have an upper respiratory disorder, treat promptly.

WHAT SHOULDN'T YOU DO?

- Don't smoke. Don't drink alcohol.
- Don't eat spicy, greasy, or fried food.

Folk Remedies

- Use your thumb and index finger to hold both top tips of the ears and pull your ears upward 100 times. Drink one cup of water. Repeat this procedure three times a day.
- Use a facial steamer and blow warm steam into your throat. It is available in the health section in many department stores.
- Before meals, use your right thumb and index finger to gently press and release continuously the tip of your left ring finger for 10 minutes, three times a day.

Food Therapy

- Take egg with sesame oil and sugar:
    Ingredients: 1 egg, 1 tsp. sesame oil, 1/2 tsp. sugar.
    Procedure: Beat an egg with sesame oil and sugar. Pour the mixture into a cup of boiling water on a pan on the stove. Cook for 40 seconds. Drink twice a day.

☞ Eat seaweed with sugar:

> **Ingredients:** 1 oz. kelp (seaweed), 1/2 oz. sugar.
>
> **Procedure:** Soak the kelp in water for three hours. Wash and clean the kelp. Slice into small pieces. Place in a pot, and add water to cover. Cook until well done. Strain water, and place the kelp in a bowl. Add sugar to marinate for one day. Eat 1 oz. at a time, twice a day.

☞ For a chronic case eat fresh water chestnut juice:

> **Ingredients:** 1.5 lb. water chestnuts, 2 oz. crystal sugar.
>
> **Procedure:** Wash and peel water chestnuts. Use a juicer to make juice. Add sugar and eat 2 oz. at a time, twice a day for three days.

☞ For a chronic case, drink watermelon peel soup. Add an adequate amount of water to cook watermelon peels. Drink it as tea.

Chinese Massage

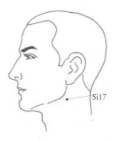
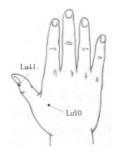

☞ Use both thumbs to gently push and knead outward from the Adam's apple to your earlobes. Pinch and knead the earlobe several times. Repeat this procedure five to ten times.

☞ Bend your index and middle fingers like forceps, and use them to gently grasp the muscles around your Adam's apple. Pull and release these muscles for one minute.

☞ Use your thumb to gently knead the point just behind the corner of the lower jaw for one minute (Si17). Repeat on opposite side.

☞ Use your right thumb to press the point on the outer lower corner of the thumbnail for one minute (Lu11). Repeat on opposite side.

☞ With your thumb against the index finger, use your other thumb to gently press and knead the webbing where it bulges up the highest for one minute (Li4).

Chinese Herbs

☞ In an acute case, squirt the patent herb powder Shuang Liao Hou Feng San into your throat, three times a day. If you have an allergic reaction stop.

☞ Drink boat sterculia seed tea:

> **Ingredients:** 4 boat sterculia seeds, 1/4 oz. ophiopogon, 1/2 oz. crystal sugar.

> **Procedure:** Place herbs in a big bowl with sugar. Add 1 cup of boiling water and cover with a lid for 30 minutes. The boat sterculia seeds will become very puffy. Discard all herbs. Drink the decoction as tea frequently.

Strain and Sprain

WHAT IS IT AND WHAT CAUSES IT?

Strain is a muscle injury caused by sudden overstretching. The symptoms are pain, swelling, or discoloration in the injured area. Sprain is an injury to the ligaments mostly caused by a sudden, forceful movement. The symptoms are joint pain or swelling with limited motion and discoloration.

WHEN SHOULD YOU SEE A DOCTOR?

If you have severe pain or have swelling, or are disfigured, go to an emergency room immediately. If you see no sign of improvement after three days self-treatment, or the condition gets worse, see a doctor.

WHAT SHOULD YOU DO IN DAILY LIFE?

☞ For the first two or three days after injury, apply ice to your joint for 15 to 20 minutes three to four times a day.

Raising the injured part above your heart would help to reduce the swelling. When the inflammation is gone, you could use a heating pad and start massage.

WHAT SHOULDN'T YOU DO?

- Don't use the injured joint if possible. Don't pull or twist the injury forcefully.
- Don't do any massage when you have a new injury.

Folk Remedies

- Fresh crab is a good sprain cure:

    Ingredients: 1/2 lb. fresh crabmeat.

    Procedure: Wash crabmeat and wrap it with a piece of clean gauze. Mash it and apply to the painful joint for one hour.

- Steam with pine dust:

    Ingredients: 1 lb. pine tree dust, 500 ml rice vinegar.

    Procedure: Place all ingredients in a large pot. Add 1 1/2 cups of water and bring to a boil. Place your injured joint 1 foot above the container. Cover the painful spot with a towel and steam for 20 minutes. Repeat twice a day for five days. Don't burn yourself.

- Apply red small bean paste for swelling:

    Ingredients: 3 oz. red small beans.

    Procedure: Grind red beans into a fine powder. Add enough water to make a paste. Apply a 1/4-inch thick paste to the injured joint. Wrap with clear plastic wrap. Change the paste every 5 hours.

Chinese Massage

Choose any combination of the following you are comfortable with. Do not massage if you have an acute injury with swelling.

- For an injury to the wrist, do the following:
    - Use your thumb to find the most painful spot, and gently press and knead it for two minutes.

☞ Rub-roll your upper arm for one minute.

☞ Use your thumb and fingers to grab the middle finger of the injured side. Gently pull outwards, then shake up and down for one minute. Repeat this for the ring finger.

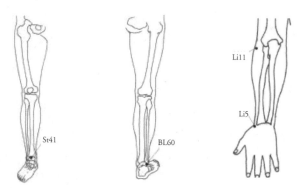

☞ Gently press and knead the point at the end of the crease on the top of the elbow joint, when the arm is folded across the chest for one minute (Li11).

☞ Gently press and knead the point on the back of the hand in the depression where the wrist crease meets the line from the thumb for one minute (Li5).

☞ Hold your injured wrist with the opposite hand and gently rotate. Bend it up several times.

☜ For an injury to the knee, see **Knee Pain** section.

☜ For an injury to the ankle, do the following:

☞ Place your leg on a low stool. Use the heel of your palm to gently rub and knead the inner and outer areas of the lower leg from top to bottom for one minute. Gradually increase the pressure.

☞ Place your foot on a low stool. Use both thumbs to gently press and knead the area surrounding the injured joint for one minute.

☞ Place your leg on a low stool. Place the thumb of each hand in the depression between the anklebone and Achilles tendon on the middle of the ankle. Push and press downwards first, then press along the lower edge of the anklebone to the front edge of the anklebone.

- ☞ Put one hand over the other and use the palm to gently press and knead the injured area for one minute.

- ☞ Use your thumb to gently press the point in the middle of the front ankle crease, level with the anklebone, for one minute (St41).

- ☞ Gently press the point in the depression behind the top of the outside anklebone for one minute (Bl60).

- ☞ If your left ankle is injured, use your left hand to hold the ankle in the front, placing your thumb and index finger on the lower edges of the anklebone. Use your right hand to hold the left foot, and gently stretch the left foot down and up as much as possible. Repeat this procedure three times. Vice versa. Stop if it is painful.

Chinese Herbs

- ☞ Take the patent herb Yu Nan Bai Yao. Or rub Yu Nan Bai Yao tincture on the injured part. Follow the instructions. If you have an allergic reaction, stop.

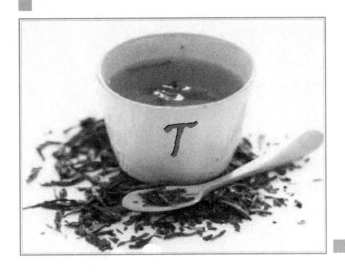

Tennis Elbow (Chronic)

WHAT IS IT AND WHAT CAUSES IT?

Tennis elbow is tendonitis. The main symptom is pain and tenderness on the inside or outside of the elbow. It is often caused by small tears in the tendons due to excessive, repeated movement or sudden twisting of the elbow.

WHEN SHOULD YOU SEE A DOCTOR?

If you have had pain for more than one week, see a doctor.

WHAT SHOULD YOU DO IN DAILY LIFE?

- Rest your arm for a while. Be patient and give it time to heal.
- Soaking your elbow in warm water for 10 minutes or applying a heating pad several times a day may help.
- Always keep your elbow warm. Cut a piece of thick fabric and sew this fabric on the sleeve of your clothes. Or cut

281

large, old socks in half and wear on your elbow during your sleep. It must be loose to increase blood circulation.

* Walking 30 minutes daily, while naturally swinging your arms, may help.

* Try wearing an elbow brace.

WHAT SHOULDN'T YOU DO?

* Don't do prolonged, repeated bending or rotating of your elbow or forearm. Always warm up your arm and wrist by stretching and flexing them. Take breaks between the activities.

Folk Remedies

* Steam with chili pepper: Place some dehydrated small chili peppers in a metal container. Burn it outside your house. Place your arm over it to steam for 10 minutes, once a day.

* Apply ginger and onion:

    Ingredients: 3 oz. prickly ash peels, 1/2 oz. fresh ginger, 6 white stalks of green onion.

    Procedure: Slice ginger into small pieces. Place all ingredients in a cotton bag. Apply the bag to your elbow for 30 minutes with a heating pad on top, twice a day for seven days. If you have an allergic reaction, stop.

* Cut old and large socks in half to fit your arm and soak in vodka. Wear on your forearm and wrap with clear plastic wrap. It must be loose to increase blood circulation. Apply a heating pad on top. Wear for 30 minutes, once a day. If you have an allergic reaction stop.

Chinese Massage

Choose the following and massage once a day:

* Using your palm very gently knead and rub the muscles around your elbow for two minutes. Using your thumb or index finger, gently press and knead the painful spot and its edges for two minutes.

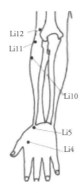 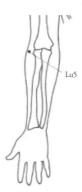

✍ Using the side of the palm on the little finger side, push the outside muscles of your upper arm down to the forearm and wrist for one minute. Using your palm, rub back and forth over the affected arm from the shoulder down to the wrist for one minute.

✍ Using your fingers and the heel of the palm, grasp your arm and massage from the shoulder to the wrist several times.

✍ Using your thumb, index, and middle fingers, grasp the following points for one minute:

☞ When your arm is folded across your chest, the point at the end of the crease on the top of the elbow joint (Li11).

☞ With your thumb against the index finger, the webbing where it bulges up the highest (Li4).

✍ Using your thumb, gently press and knead the following points for one minute, while bending and stretching your forearm:

☞ When the arm is folded across the chest, the point at the end of the crease on the top of the elbow joint (Li11).

☞ The point two thumb-widths down below Li11 point (Li10).

☞ The point one thumb's-width above Li11 (Li12).

☞ The point on the inside crease of the elbow in the depression on the outer edge of the tendon (Lu5).

☞ On the back of the hand in the depression, where the wrist crease meets the line from the thumb (Li5).

Chinese Herbs

☜ Apply a heating patch with herb, called Chinese Moxibustion. Follow the instructions.

☜ Apply the herb patch Shang Shi Zhi Tong Gao. If you have an allergic reaction, stop.

TMD (Temporomandibular Disorder)

WHAT IS IT AND WHAT CAUSES IT?

Temporomandibular disorder was formerly called "temporomandibular joint syndrome" (TMJ). The symptom is a painful jaw with difficulty chewing and talking. Emotional stress is the most common cause of TMD.

WHEN SHOULD YOU SEE A DOCTOR?

If you have persistent pain in your jaw, see a doctor.

WHAT SHOULD YOU DO IN DAILY LIFE?

↝ Rest your jaw as much as possible.

↝ Keep warm always.

↝ When you have an acute attack, apply ice for 15 minutes to relieve the pain and reduce the swelling, three times a day. In a chronic case, apply a heating pad to increase local blood circulation.

↝ Eat soft food.

↝ Reduce stress as much as you can.

WHAT SHOULDN'T YOU DO?

↝ Don't sleep on your stomach with your head twisted to one side. Don't read a book with your head propped up on a pillow at a sharp angle. Avoid activities that twist, bend, or raise your head for a prolonged period.

Don't cradle the phone between your neck and shoulder. Don't carry a heavy bag on your shoulder.

* Don't open your mouth too wide while yawning.
* Don't chew gum. Avoid hard, crunchy food.
* Don't expose yourself to wind. Wear a mask or scarf in cold weather.

Chinese Massage

Choose the following and massage each point for one to two minutes, once a day:

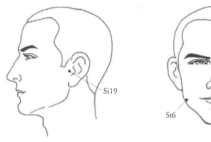 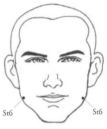 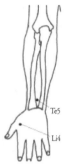

* Use the pad of your thumb to find the painful point on the lower jaw. Gently press and knead that point. Flick the muscles several times.
* Use your thumb to push from the indentation level with the top of the ear down to the lower jawbone.
* Use your thumb to gently press and knead the depression in front of the middle of the ear when the mouth is slightly open (Si19).
* Use your thumb to gently press and knead the point in the corner of the lower jawbone, in the high point formed by the muscles when the teeth are clenched (St6). Open and close your mouth while massaging this point.
* With your thumb against the index finger, use your other thumb to gently press and knead the webbing where it bulges up the highest (Li4).

↝ Gently press and knead the point two thumb-widths above the wrist in the depression between the bones on the back of the forearm (Te5).

Toothache

WHAT IS IT AND WHAT CAUSES IT?

Toothache is a commonly encountered problem. The main cause of toothache is tooth decay, which can lead to infection in the root of your tooth.

WHEN SHOULD YOU SEE A DOCTOR?

If you have a toothache, see your dentist.

WHAT SHOULD YOU DO IN DAILY LIFE?

↝ Rinse vigorously with a mouthful of warm, salty water. Or swish your mouth with liquor, but don't drink the alcohol. Swish 3-percent hydrogen peroxide solution in your mouth for five seconds and spit out.

↝ Ice your cheek with a frozen vegetable bag or a reusable gel pack wrapped with thin cloth for 10 minutes. Apply a warm, wet black tea bag.

↝ Eat more pumpkins, watermelon, water chestnuts, celery, and daikon radish.

↝ Have regular bowel movements.

↝ Control your emotions, which may be a trigger for tooth pain.

↝ Use special toothpaste for sensitive teeth.

↝ Be aware that trigeminal neuralgia and temporomandibular disorder will cause tooth pain.

WHAT SHOULDN'T YOU DO?

↝ Don't eat food that is too cold, too hot, or too sour. Don't eat spicy food such as onions, mustard, and chili peppers.

Folk Remedies

- ☙ Chewing soaked green tea leaves may give some relief.
- ☙ Rinse your mouth with vinegar and prickly ash peels:

    Ingredients: 60 ml rice vinegar, 60 ml water, 1 oz. prickly ash peels.

    Procedure: Boil ingredients in a pot on low heat for 10 minutes. Wait until it cools. Rinse your mouth for two minutes and spit out. Then wash your mouth with warm water. Don't swallow.

Food Therapy

- ☙ Drink tofu soup with olives:

    Ingredients: 4 salty olives, 1 lb. tofu.

    Procedure: Add 2 cups of water to make soup. Eat once a day.

Chinese Massage

In general, choose the following to get some relief.

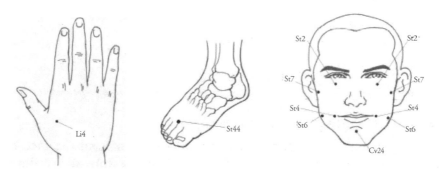

- ☙ With your thumb against the index finger, use your hand to pinch the webbing where it bulges up the highest (Li4). If the painful tooth is on the left, pinch the opposite hand. Vice versa.

☞ Press and knead the point on the base of toes between the second toe and the third toe (St44).

Specially for an upper tooth:

☞ Gently press and knead the depression in front of the ear while the mouth is closed (St7). The depression disappears when the mouth is open.

☞ Using both index fingers, gently press the point one finger's-width right below the eye socket in line with the pupil (St2).

Specially for a lower tooth:

☞ Using your thumb, gently press the point in the corner of the lower jawbone, in the high point formed by the muscles when the teeth are clenched (St6).

☞ Using both index fingers, gently press and knead the points at the corners of the mouth as it is closed (St4). Gently press and knead the depression in the center of the groove between the chin and lower lip (Cv24).

Chinese Herbs

☞ Spread the patent herb powder Yun Nan Bai Yao on the painful spot. Follow the instructions.

Trigeminal Neuralgia

WHAT IS IT AND WHAT CAUSES IT?

Trigeminal nerves convey sensory information from the face to the brain. A disruption of their functions, such as pressure from a blood vessel, can cause the brief but excruciating, stabbing pain on one side of the face, which is the symptom of trigeminal neuralgia.

WHEN SHOULD YOU SEE A DOCTOR?

If you have persistent face pain and no sign of improvement, see a doctor.

WHAT SHOULD YOU DO IN DAILY LIFE?

- When you have pain, soak your feet in warm water at a temperature you can tolerate. Meanwhile, massage the sole of your foot and the area around the anklebone. Soaking your feet in warm water frequently can reduce the chance of an attack.

- When you are washing your face, brushing your teeth, or eating, do so very gently. Sometimes, daily activities such as brushing your teeth can trigger an episode. Don't use water that is too hot or too cold.

WHAT SHOULDN'T YOU DO?

- Don't eat spicy or greasy food, hot pepper, curry, ginger powder, or mustard. Eat soft food only. Avoid crab, shrimp, and other seafood, fried foods and nuts.

- Don't drink alcohol or coffee. Do not consume food or liquids that are too hot.

- Don't smoke. Nicotine will contract the blood vessels and trigger the pain.

- Don't expose yourself to wind. Wear a scarf over your face in cold weather.

- Limit stress both mentally and physically. Stress may be the most common trigger.

Folk Remedies

- Comb your head with a wooden comb: Comb from your forehead to the top then down the back of your head 20 times per minute. You can increase the speed gradually. Comb evenly with adequate force, but not too hard to damage your skin. Comb for five minutes every time. Repeat this procedure three times a day for one month. This procedure is good for first branch nerve pain.

- Drop radish juice in the nose. Use a juicer to make red radish juice. Lie down on your back. Use an eyedropper and apply two drops in the nostril on the side of the facial pain.

Food Therapy

☞ Drink sunflower petal tea:

Ingredients: 4 oz. sunflower petal (dried, without seeds), 2 Tbs. sugar.

Procedure: Wash the petal clean. Cut into small pieces and put in a pot with 4 cups of water. Bring to a boil. Reduce heat and simmer for 15 minutes. Strain the decoction into a container. Then start a second batch. Add 2 cups of water into the pot and follow the above instructions to make another decoction. Mix the two decoctions together. Drink 100 ml one hour after meals, twice a day for five days. Keep unused decoction in a refrigerator.

Chinese Massage

Choose the following and massage once a day:

☞ Rub both palms against each other until they feel warm. Place them on your face and rub gently up and down 30 times. Don't touch the area that triggers the pain.

☞ Gently press and knead the temples with your fingers until you have a sensation of soreness and distention.

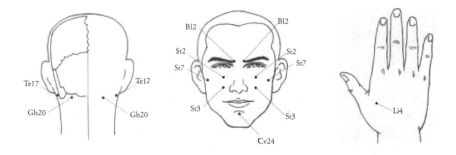

☞ Gently press and knead the point in the depression at the bottom of the skull, outside of the two big muscles on the neck, which you can feel by bending down your neck for two minutes (Gb20).

- Use your thumb to gently press the depression in front of the ear while the mouth is closed (St7). The depression disappears when the mouth is open. At the same time, use your index fingers to gently press the depression directly behind the earlobe (Te17). Gently press these points simultaneously for one minute.

- With your thumb against the index finger, use your other thumb to gently press and knead the webbing where it bulges up the highest (Li4).

- If you have forehead pain, gently press and knead the point in the depression on the beginning of the eyebrow for one minute (Bl2).

- If you have pain from the upper jaw, gently press and knead the following points for one minute:
  - The point one finger's-width right below the eye socket, in line with the pupil (St2).
  - The point on the cheek directly under the eye pupil and level with the low edge of the nostril (St3).

- If you have pain from the lower jaw, gently press and knead the following points for one minute:
  - The depression in the center of the groove between the chin and lower lip (Cv24).
  - The depression in front of the ear while the mouth is closed (St7). The depression disappears when the mouth is open.

Chinese Herbs

- Steam your face with herbs:

  Ingredients: 1/4 oz. siler, 1/4 oz. notopterygium root, 1/4 oz. dang gui, 1/4 oz. ligusticum, 1/4 oz. batryticated silkworm.

  Procedure: Add ingredients to 4 cups of water. Bring to a boil. Reduce heat and simmer for 20 minutes. Steam your face for 20 minutes, twice a day. Be careful not to scald your face.

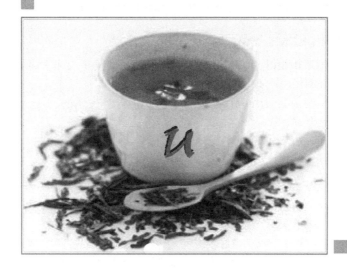

Urinary Incontinence

WHAT IS IT AND WHAT CAUSES IT?

It is the inability of the bladder to hold urine. The urine is released with any movement that adds pressure to the belly. Along with aging, urinary incontinence can be caused by some medications, urinary tract infections, nerve damage, prostate problems for men, and weakened muscles of the pelvic floor for women after childbirth.

WHEN SHOULD YOU SEE A DOCTOR?

If you experience an abrupt loss of bladder control or your incontinence interferes with your daily life, see a doctor.

WHAT SHOULD YOU DO IN DAILY LIFE?

- Set a regular schedule to go to the bathroom, whether or not you have to go. Spend more time in the bathroom and try to totally empty your bladder. Then gradually increase the interval between bathroom visits.
- Drink normally, but control fluid intake at night. Be sure to urinate before bedtime.

➻ If you know the kind of situation that will cause loss of bladder control, such as laughing, coughing or sneezing, cross your legs before to avoid any accident.

WHAT SHOULDN'T YOU DO?

➻ Limit drinking alcohol, coffee, soda, or tea, all of which can stimulate urination.

➻ Don't use artificial sweeteners, as they can irritate the bladder.

Folk Remedies

➻ If you feel you are on the verge of losing bladder control, stay calm and keep still. Use your thumb to gently press and knead the point four finger-widths up from the inside anklebone, right behind the leg bone (Sp6). When the urge subsides, slowly go to the restroom.

➻ Put some black pepper powders in a little bag made from thin cotton fabric and apply to your belly button. Use a bandage to fix, and sleep with it. Repeat once a day for one week. If you have an allergic reaction on the skin, stop.

➻ Eat egg with white peppercorn: Open a small hole in an uncooked egg. Insert five white peppercorn and seal with paper. Steam until well done. Cook two daily and eat them before bedtime without water for one week.

➻ Rub with liquor soaked with ginger:

Ingredients: 1 oz. ginger, 100 ml 80-proof vodka.

Procedure: Smash the ginger and soak it in vodka. Before bedtime, dab a piece of gauze in the vodka and rub your midline right below the bellybutton for one minute. Repeat nightly for five days. If you have an allergic reaction, stop.

Food Therapy

➻ Eat walnuts, red dates, and sesame seeds:

Ingredients: 1/2 oz. walnuts, 1/4 oz. black sesame seeds, 5 red dates without the kernel.

Procedure: Stir-fry walnuts and sesame seeds on low heat until light brown. Crush and eat twice a day.

☞ Eat dry litchi (Asian fruit): Eat 10 dry litchis daily for one week.

☞ Drink corn silk tea: Place 1 oz. of corn silk in 2 cups of water in a pot. Bring to a boil. Reduce heat and simmer for 10 minutes. Add 1 Tbs. of sugar and drink once a day for one week.

Chinese Massage

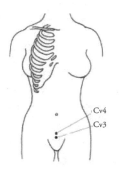
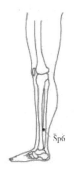
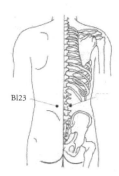

☞ Use your thumb to gently press and knead the point four finger-widths up from the inside anklebone, right behind the leg bone for two minutes (Sp6).

☞ Use your thumb to gently press and knead the point on the midline of the lower abdomen, about one hand's-width below the belly button for one minute (Cv3).

☞ Use your thumb to gently press and knead the point on the midline of the abdomen four finger-widths below the belly button for one minute (Cv4).

☞ Use your thumb and other fingers to grasp the muscles right below your belly button 10 times. Use your palm to gently rub your belly button counterclockwise until it feels warm.

☞ Use the pad of the heel of your palm to gently press and knead the points a little higher than the waist, two finger-widths on both sides of the spine for one minute (Bl23).

Heat Therapy

Light a smokeless moxa stick, which is like a cigar and available in Chinese herb stores. Circle it 1 to 2 inches above the midpoint between the bellybutton and pubic bone for 10 minutes. Repeat one or two times a day. Be careful not to let the stick or its ashes burn you.

Chinese Herbs

☞ Take the patent herb Bu Zhong Yi Qi Wan. Follow the instructions.

Urinary Tract Calculus (Kidney Stone)

WHAT IS IT AND WHAT CAUSES IT?

It is a mineral substance formation in the kidney, ureter, urethra, or bladder due to concentrated urine that cannot contribute enough fluid to flush those substances away. When a large stone travels down, it can cause excruciating pain in your back or side. As the stone continues to move down, the pain also moves down. Other symptoms are bloody urine, urge to urinate, failure to empty the bladder, vomiting, fever, or chills.

The following remedies are not for you if you have urinary tract obstruction. If the size of stone is less than a 1/4 inch with a round and smooth surface with no severe blockage of the urinary tract, you can choose a conservative therapy.

WHEN SHOULD YOU SEE A DOCTOR?

When urinating, if you experience pain and perhaps a burning sensation, nausea, vomiting, or have a fever, see a doctor.

WHAT SHOULD YOU DO IN DAILY LIFE?

⚹ Drink at least 3 quarts of water daily to flush the small stones into the bladder. In order to maintain adequate hydration and urination, drink water before bedtime, and even at midnight.

- Save your urine in a clear plastic bottle, so you can see whether the stone has come out. Use a piece of gauze or a strainer with a fine mesh to filter out the stone. Give them to your doctor to analyze. Depending on what kind of stone you have, you should avoid specific types of foods.

- Take warm baths more frequently to help pass the stones. You can also apply a heating pad on the kidney area for 10 minutes. If you have heart problems, do not use this method.

- Eat more kiwi, Chinese black fungus, corn, walnuts, and bottle gourd (a kind of Asian vegetable).

- According to your constitution, jog, dance, or skip rope to accelerate passing the stone.

WHAT SHOULDN'T YOU DO?

- Depending on what kind of stone you have, avoid or eat less of the following foods:

  - If you have an oxalic acid stone, limit your intake of oxalate-rich foods such as spinach, rhubarb, cheese, peanut butter, nuts, beer, tea, and chocolate.

  - If you have a phosphatic acid stone, limit your intake of calcium and phosphor-rich foods such as dairy products, beans, sardines, or eel.

  - If you have a uric acid stone, limit your intake of purine-rich foods such as animal organs, beef, pork, lamb, onion, garlic, spinach, coffee, coca, strong tea, and alcohol.

- Avoid fast food and canned soup, as their sodium content is high. Avoid anything spicy such as garlic, hot peppers, onions, curry, and pepper. Avoid potatoes, soybeans, yam, cabbage, or milk, which produce more gas to add pressure to your abdominal cavity.

- Reduce your intake of sugar.

Folk Remedies

☞ Corn ears tea:

Ingredients: 2 corn ears with the kernels removed.

Procedure: Wash corn ears well. Cut them into small pieces. Steep with boiling water. Cover with a lid. Drink when it becomes cool twice a day for a week. If you have corn silk, that is even better.

☞ Yellow croaker:

Ingredients: 1 yellow croaker (a kind of fish, available in Chinese seafood grocery stores), salt.

Procedure: Take two white, stone-like bones from the craoker's head (called Fish Head Stone). Bake it until dry and grind into a fine powder. Take with warm water. Add water to make fish soup with the rest of the fish. Add salt. Eat the fish and drink the soup.

Food Therapy

☞ Walnuts with sugar:

Ingredients: 3 oz. walnuts, 3 oz. sugar, 120 ml. sesame oil.

Procedure: Stir-fry walnuts in sesame oil until crunchy. Grind walnuts with sugar into a fine powder. Mix with some sesame oil, and take twice a day.

☞ Chinese black fungus:

Ingredients: Chinese black fungus, Chinese cabbage, carrots, salt, vegetable oil.

Procedure: Soak black fungus in water for two hours. Stir-fry all ingredients. Take two times a day for two weeks.

☞ Eat pumpkin seeds. Eat pumpkin frequently.

☞ Eat chicken's gizzard skin with pearl barley:

Ingredients: 1/4 oz. chicken's gizzard skin (available in Chinese herb stores), 2 oz. Chinese pearl barley, 2 Tbs. brown sugar.

Procedure: Place ingredients in a pot and add 2 cups of water to make a soup. Drink once a day. Chicken's gizzard skin is a special cure for urinary tract stones.

Chinese Massage

Massage the following to get some relief:

☞ Sit on a chair. Rub your palms against each other until

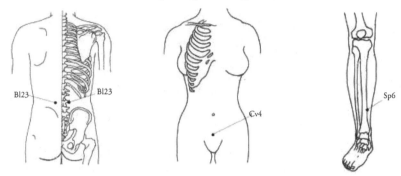

they become warm. Use your palms to rub your lower back to the sacral bone until it becomes warm.

☞ Make fists. Use the knuckles of both your hands to press and knead the points a little higher than the waist, two finger-widths on both sides of the spine for one minute (Bl23).

☞ Place the center of your left palm on the point three finger-widths down below the belly button. Gently press and knead clockwise 30 times. Use the tip of your thumb to gently press the point on the midline of the abdomen four finger-widths below the belly button (Cv4).

☞ Use four fingers of your left hand and push from inner side of the left knee to the top of the thigh 30 times. Repeat on the right side.

☞ Use the tips of both thumbs to gently press and knead the point four finger-widths up from the inside ankle-bone, right behind the leg bone for one minute (Sp6).

Chinese Herbs

☞ Take the patent herb Jin Qian Chao Chong Ji. Follow the instructions.

Urinary Tract Infection (UTI)

WHAT IS IT AND WHAT CAUSES IT?

A UTI is caused by a bacterial infection in the urethra. This condition is much more common in women due to the shorter length of their urinary tracts. Common symptoms include intense pain, smelly urine, and a frequent urge to urinate.

WHEN SHOULD YOU SEE A DOCTOR?

If you are experiencing the above symptoms, see a doctor.

WHAT SHOULD YOU DO IN DAILY LIFE?

* Drink a lot of water and cranberry juice. Eat more vegetables and fruits.
* Wash the genital area in the shower, not by taking a bath.
* Whatever method you use, if you are feeling better, you should still continue the treatment for three more days. Don't stop too early.
* In chronic cases you should also limit sexual contact, and have your partner tested for bacteria. Both participants should wash the genital area before sex.

WHAT SHOULDN'T YOU DO?

* Don't use basic soap. It neutralizes the acidic environment of the urinary tract, which is needed to fight off bacteria.
* If you have an acute UTI, you should not have sex.
* Don't eat overstimulating foods such as spicy or fried food. Don't drink alcohol or coffee.
* Don't wear tight underwear and pants.

Folk Remedies

* Boil 2 oz. of corn silk in water and drink as tea, three times a day.
* Boil watermelon peels as tea, and drink 8 cups a day.

☞ Crush one handful of white stalks of green onion. Place them in a thin cotton bag. Apply to your belly button, and tape. If you have an allergic reaction, stop.

Food Therapy

☞ Make fresh celery juice with a juicer. Drink 50 ml at a time, three times a day.

☞ Peel 8 oz. of loofah (silk melon, available in Chinese grocery stores). Boil with 2 cups of water. Drink a cup every morning and night.

☞ Cook 2 oz. of millet with water to make soup. Drink three times a day for 10 days. After that, reduce to 1 oz. of millet and continue for an additional 10 days.

Chinese Massage

Choose the following and massage each for one or two minutes:

☞ Place your right palm below your belly button. Overlap with your left palm. Gently press and knead clockwise.

☞ Place your palm on the midline of the chest. Gently push down to the pubic area. Gradually increase the pressure as long as it feels comfortable.

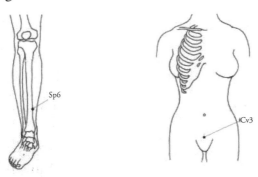

☞ Lay down on a bed. Bend your knees and raise both thighs. Use your thumb and four fingers to gently grasp the muscles on the lower abdomen several times.

- ☞ If you have painful spots on your inner thigh, use your thumb to gently press these spots several times.
- ☞ Place the pad of your thumbs on both sides of the spine. Rub the waist down to the sacrum area.
- ☞ Gently press and knead the point four finger-widths from the inside anklebone, right behind the leg bone (Sp6).
- ☞ Gently press and knead the point on the midline of the lower abdomen, about one hand's-width below the belly button (Cv3).

Chinese Herbs

- ☞ Take the patent herb Ba Zheng San. Follow the instructions.

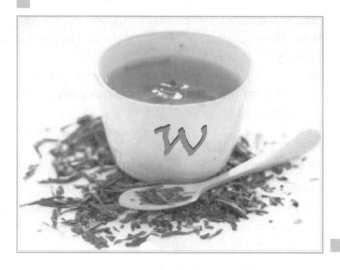

Weight Control

WHAT IS IT AND WHAT CAUSES IT?

Losing weight has always been a favorite New Year's resolution. But keeping the weight off is a problem that's not so easily solved. Yet weight control is a health issue and can be treated. Keep your goal in mind and your patient and persistent effort will bear fruit.

WHEN SHOULD YOU SEE A DOCTOR?

You may need to consult with your doctor about your weight loss program to be sure that the plan fits your physical and health conditions.

WHAT SHOULD YOU DO IN DAILY LIFE?

- Set up an exercise schedule and stick to it. At least walk whenever possible. Resist the temptation to make excuses to stop exercising, as once you stop, it is difficult to continue.
- Control your diet. Eat less but have more meals each day. Drink soup before you have meals. In this way you won't feel hungry. Eat less sugary, salty, and fried food.

303

Add rice vinegar to your diet. The amino acid in the vinegar can transfer your fat to energy and accelerate metabolism. Eat more garlic, cabbage, carrots, celery, tomatoes, cucumber, soybeans, taro root, apples, papaya, oranges, bean sprouts, or winter melon. They are called "lose-weight" food.

↳ No matter what methods you use to lose weight, you need to be persistent and apply the methods over a long period of time.

WHAT SHOULDN'T YOU DO?

↳ Don't drink alcohol, which is high in calories. Avoid over-stimulating food such as spicy foods, or caffeine.

↳ Don't eat too much at dinnertime, because people tend to be less active at night and, therefore, have less opportunity to burn off the calories.

↳ Don't stop eating or drastically reduce your food intake in order to lose weight. A gradual weight loss is much more healthy than a sudden weight loss.

Folk Remedies

☞ Bathe with herbs: With enough water, boil together 1 lb. of winter melon peels, 10 oz. of poria peels, and 4 oz. of papaya. Discard the solids and add the decoction to your bathwater. Bathe once a day for a month.

☞ Exercise by jumping rope or climbing stairs daily for a prolonged period. If you climb stairs for 10 minutes, the calories you burn are much more than those burned by walking. You can see your waist size reduce.

☞ Take warm and cold showers alternately. Start with warm water, then switch to cold water. Repeat three times. Finish with warm water. Don't get cold.

Food Therapy

☞ Eat cooked bananas:

Ingredients: 1 ripe banana.

Procedure: Peel banana. Cut into pieces. Place them in a pan with 1 cup of water. Bring to boil. Simmer for 10 minutes. Eat one banana a day for a prolonged period.

☞ Drink lotus leaf soup:

Ingredients: 1/8 oz. dry lotus leaves (available in Chinese grocery stores).

Procedure: Clean the lotus leaves first. Soak them overnight in water. Cut them into pieces. Add 2 cups of water. Bring to a boil. Reduce heat and simmer for 10 minutes. Divide into two portions for two days. Drink three times a day. Warm it before drinking.

☞ Drink red small bean soup:

Ingredients: 2 oz. Red small beans.

Procedure: Soak beans in 4 cups water overnight. Bring to a boil. Reduce heat and simmer for an hour. Drink 100 ml each time, three times a day.

☞ Drink a mixture of 1 Tbs. rice vinegar, 1/2 Tbs. honey, and 3 Tbs. of warm water every day.

Chinese Massage

☞ Before getting up in the morning and after going to bed at night, do the following massage once a day:

⮞ Place your right palm on your bellybutton and your left on top of the right. Rub your abdomen outward in a counterclockwise direction 100 times.

⮞ Put the left palm on the bottom and start from the outer edge of the abdomen and rub inward in a clockwise direction. Repeat on opposite side.

⮞ Place your palms on the abdomen area, push down to pubic area 100 times.

⮞ Place your right palm on the lower edge of right ribs. Push toward left groin area 50 times. Repeat on the other side.

☙ Finally, press and knead your arms and legs for 10 minutes.

☙ Prepare a long towel. Put cornstarch or massage oil on your waist to protect your skin. Your waist should be bare. Stand with feet shoulder width apart and wrap the towel around the back of your waist. Hold the two ends of the towel in your hands and pull it back and forth so it scrapes across your waist. Do so until you feel heat and the skin is flush.

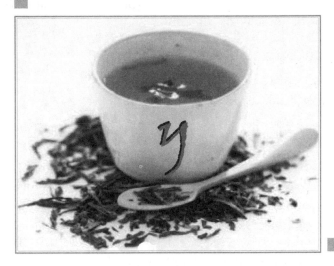

Yeast Infections

WHAT IS IT AND WHAT CAUSES IT?

Yeast infections are caused by the rampant growth of a fungus in and around the vagina. Although the fungus is a normal inhabitant, certain environmental factors, such as hormone imbalance and antibiotics, may trigger its uncontrolled growth. Yeast infections are characterized by an itching, burning sensation with a smelly discharge.

WHEN SHOULD YOU SEE A DOCTOR?

If self-treatment is not working or you have had recurrent yeast infections, see a doctor.

WHAT SHOULD YOU DO IN DAILY LIFE?

* Try to determine conditions that trigger the infections, such as preexisting diabetes. Consult with your doctor to see if you are taking too much antibiotics.
* Change your cotton underwear often, and disinfect the used underwear and towels. Or don't wear undwear at all becasue yeast loves warm and moist places.

- Increase water intake.
- If you have a partner, both of you need to clean the genital area before sex. After that you should urinate to dilute the basicity of semen.

WHAT SHOULDN'T YOU DO?

- Don't eat too much sugar or spicy food.
- Don't drink alcohol.

Folk Remedies

- Wash with vinegar and prickly ash peel:

    Ingredients: 5 prickly ash peel, 150 ml dark rice vinegar, 500 ml water.

    Procedure: After boiling wait until cool, then wash the genital area every night. Do a skin test first. If you have an allergic reaction, stop.

- Apply plain yogurt in and around your vagina. Wash thoroughly after 20 minutes. Repeat twice a day for a week. Yogurt can restrain yeast overgrowth.

Food Therapy

- Eat garlic salad: Smash a clove of garlic. Mix with 1/4 tsp. and 1 Tbs. olive iol. Use as salad dressing on your favorite vegetables. Eat twice a day. If stomach feels uncomfortable, discontinue use.
- Eat 5 Tbs. plain yogurt, three times a day.

Chinese Herbs

- Wash with herb decoction:

    Ingredients: 1/2 oz. bitter ginseng, 1/2 oz. cnidium fruit, 1/2 oz. smilax glabra rhizome, 1/4 oz. phellodendron bark, 1/4 oz. prickly ash peel.

    Procedure: Add ingredients to 4 cups of water and bring to a boil. Reduce heat and simmer for 20 minutes. Wait until cool and wash your genital area once a day. Do a skin test first. If you have an allergic reaction, discontinue use.

Appendix

Chinese Herbs and Asian Food List

Common Name	English Spelling of Chinese
American Ginseng	Xi Yang Shen
Angelica root	Bai Zhi
Apricot seed	Xing Ren
Astragalus root	Huang Qi
Batryticated Silkworm	Jiang Can
Bitter melon (bitter gourd)	Ku Gua
Black dates	Hei Zao
Black plum	Wu Mei
Bok Choy	Shanghai Xiao Bai Cai
Borneol	Bing Pian
Boat sterculia seed	Pang Da Hai
Bupleurum	Chai Hu
Chinese Moxibustion	Zhong Hua Jiou
Chinese okra	Si Gua
Chicken's gizzard skin	Ji Nei Jin

Common Name	English Spelling of Chinese
Chinese dried mushroom	Xiang Gu
Chinese black fungus	Hei Mu Er
Chinese white fungus	Bai Mu Er
Chinese rose flower	Yue Ji Hua
Chinese pearl barley	Yi Yi Ren
Chinese chives	Jiu Cai
Chinese mustard seed	Jie Cai Zi
Chinese mustard leaf	Jie Cai
Chinese yam	Shan Yao
Chrysanthemum	Ju Hua
Cinnamon twig	Gui Zhi
Citrus	Chen Pi
Cnidium fruit	She Chung Zi
Codonopsis	Dang Shen
Cooked rehmannia	Shu Di Huang
Corn silk (Corn stigma)	Yu Mi Xu
Crucian carp	Ji Yu
Crystal sugar	Bing Tang
Curculigo rhizome	Xian Mao
Dang Gui	Dang Gui
Dandelion	Pu Gong Ying
Gardenia fruit	Zhi Zi
Daylily (Gold needle vegetable)	Huang Hua Cai
Deer pilose antler	Lu Rong
Deglued antler powder	Lu Jiao Shuang
Dogbane	Lo Bu Ma
Donkey-hide gelatin	A Jao
Dried ginger	Gan Jiang
Dried white bean (Dolichos seed)	Bai Pian Dou
Dogwood	Shan Zhu Yu
Dried black bean	Dou Chi
Earthworm	Di Long
Eel	Shan Yu
Epimedium	Yin Yang Huo

Common Name	English Spelling of Chinese
Fennel fruit	Xiao Hui Xiang
Fleece flower root (processed)	He Shou
Ganoderma	Ling Zhi
Gastrodia tuber	Tian Ma
Gecko	Ge Jie
Ginseng	Ren Shen
Gypsum	Shi Gao
Hawthorn fruit	Shan Zha
Honeysuckle flower	Jin Yin Hua
Houttuynia	Yu Xing Cao
IIsatis leaf	Da Qing Ye
Isatis root	Ban Lang Gen
Kelp (Seaweed)	Hai Dai
Licorice	Gan Cao
Lavender oil	Xun Yi Cao
Ligusticum	Chuan Xiong
Litchi (Lychee)	Li Che
Lily bulb	Bai He
Longan aril	Long Yan Rou
Loofah (Silk melon)	Si Gua
Loquat leaf	Pi Pa Ye
Lotus leaf	Lian Ye
Lotus node	Ou Jie
Lotus seeds	Lian Zi
Lotus flower	Lian Hua
Lucid ganoderma	Ling Zhi
Lycium fruit	Gou Ji Zi
Mastic	Ru Xiang
Menthae	Bo He
Millettia stem	Ji Xue Teng
Moutan bark	Mu Dan Pi
Mulberry	Sang Shen
Mung bean	Lu Dou
Mugwort leaf	Ai Ye

Common Name	English Spelling of Chinese
Notopterygium root	Qiang Huo
Ophiopogon	Mai Men Dong
Oriental arborvitae leaves	Ce Bai Ye
Papaya	Mu Gua
Phellodendron bark	Huang Bai
Pine nut seed	Song Zi Ren
Pilose deer horn	Lu Rong
Poria	Fu Ling
Poria peel	Fu Ling Pi
Prickly ash peel	Hua Jiao
Pseudoginseng	San Qi
Pseudostellaria root	Tai Zi Shen
Pubescent angelica root	Du Huo
Pueraria root	Ge Gen
Purslane	Ma Chi Xian
Quail egg	An Chun
Red dates	Hong Zao
Red rice yeast	Hong Qu Mei
Red peony	Chi Shao
Red small bean	Chi Xiao Dou
Rehmannia root (fresh)	Sheng Di Huang
Royal jelly	Feng Huang Jianghh
Safflower	Hong Hua
Saffron	Fan Hong Hua
Salvia root	Dan Shen
Seahorse	Hai Mal
Senna Leaf	Fan Xie Ye
Siberian ginseng	Ci Wu Jia
Siberian olomonseal rhizome	Huang Jing
Siler	Fang Feng
Smilax	Tu Fu Ling
Sophora flower	Huai Hua
Talc	Hua Shi
Tangerine peels	Chen Pi

Common Name	English Spelling of Chinese
Tato root	Yu Tou
Tendrilled fritillary bulb	Chuan Bei Mu
Thunbery fritillary bulb	Zhe Bei Mu
Tree seed oil	Cha Hua Zi You
Water spinach	Kong Xin Cai
White atractylodes	Bai Zhu
Wild rice stem	Jiao Bai
Wolfberry bark	Di Gu Pi
White peony	Bai Shao
Wild chrysanthemum flower	Ye Ju Hua
Winter melon	Dong Gua
Yellow croaker	Huang Hua Yu
Zizyphus	Suan Zao Ren

Chinese Patent Herbs

Ba Zheng San	Gu Ci Wan
Bao He Wan	Gui Pi Wan
Bi Min Gan Wan	Gu Zhi Zeng Sheng Wan
Bi Yan Pian	Huo Xiang Zheng Qi Shui
Bu Zhong Yi Qi Wan	Jiao Gu Lan Tea
Chai Hu Shu Gan Wan	Jin Gui Shen Qi Wan
Dan Zhi Xiao Yao Wan	Jin Qian Cao Chong Ji
Dang Gui Long Hui Wan	Ju He Wan
Dang Gui Wan	Kang Gu Ci Zeng Sheng Wan
Di Yu Huai Jiao Wan	Liu Shen Wan
Du Huo Ji Sheng Wan	Liu Wei Di Huang Wan
Er Chen Wan	Ma Ren Run Chang Wan
Er Long Zuo Ci Wan	Ma Ying Long Ointment
Er Miao Wan	Mei Bao
Fu Zi Li Zhong Wan	Mu Gua Wan
Gan Mao Qing Re Chong Ji	Nan Bao

Niu Huang Jiang Ya Wan
Pi Pa Ye Gao
Shang Shi Zhi Tong Gao
She Dan Chuan Bei Ye
Shen Ling Bai Zhu Wan
Shen Qi Wan
Shi Qaun Da Bu Wan
Shuang Liao Hou Feng San
Smokeless moxa stick
Tiger balm
Tong Jing Wan
Tong Xuang Li Fei Wan
Wu Ji Bai Feng Wan

Wu Shao She Pia
Vine Essence Pill
Xiao Yao Wan
Xiang Sha Liu Jun Zi Wan
Xiang Sha Yang Wei Wan
Yang Yin Qing Fei Wan
Yi Guan Jian
Yin Qiao Jie Du Pian
Yu Nan Bai Yao
Zheng Gu Shui
Zhi Bai Di Huang Wan
Zuo Jin Wan

Quick Measurement Conversion Guide

473 ml   =   1 pint for liquid measure.
240 ml   =   1 cup (some texts say 300ml = 1 cup)
1000 ml   =   4 cups.
1 Tbs.   =   15 ml,
1 shot   =   30 ml.
1 tsp.   =   5 ml.

Index

G

H

About the Author

Lihua Wang acquired formal medical education in both traditional Chinese medicine and Western medicine at Beijing University of Traditional Chinese Medicine in the People's Republic of China. Later on she began her career as a cardiologist in Xi Yuan Hospital affiliated with the China Academy of Traditional Chinese Medicine, where she practiced integrative medicine, combining both Western and Traditional Chinese Medicine. In 1982 she was invited by Kaiser Permanente Research Center as a visiting scholar. After returning to China and practicing for a while, she was invited by the Oregon College of Oriental Medicine to teach acupuncture and Chinese herbology to American students for four years before starting her private practice in Traditional Chinese Medicine in 1992 in Portland, Oregon.